Jill Weisenberger, MS, RDN, CDE, FAND

THE
OVERWORKED
PERSON'S
Guide to
BETTER
Nutrition

Simple Steps *You* Can Take to Eat Well,
Reduce Stress, and Improve Your Health

Director, Book Publishing, Abe Ogden; *Managing Editor,* Greg Guthrie; *Acquisitions Editor,* Victor Van Beuren; *Project Manager,* Wendy Martin-Shuma; *Production Manager,* Melissa Sprott; *Cover and Page Design,* Jenn French Designs, LLC; *Illustrations,* Pam Little; *Printer,* Versa Press.

Printed in the United States of America
1 3 5 7 9 10 8 6 4 2

ADA titles may be purchased for business or promotional use or for special sales. To purchase more than 50 copies of this book at a discount, or for custom editions of this book with your logo, contact the American Diabetes Association at the address below or at booksales@diabetes.org.

American Diabetes Association
1701 North Beauregard Street
Alexandria, Virginia 22311

DOI: 10.2337/9781580405416

Library of Congress Cataloging-in-Publication Data
Weisenberger, Jill.
The overworked persons guide to better nutrition : simple steps you can take to eat well, reduce stress, and improve your health / Jill Weisenberger, MS, RDN, CDE.
pages cm
Includes bibliographical references and index.
ISBN 978-1-58040-541-6 (alk. paper)
1. Health. 2. Nutrition. 3. Home economics. 4. Quick and easy cooking. 5. Stress management. I. Title.
RA776.5.W439 2014
613--dc23
2014001046

Table of Contents

Chapter 6: Beyond Food p. 113

Additional Reading p. 129

Appendix p. 131

Index p. 140

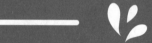

Acknowledgments

This book came to be because of the loving support and patience of my family, the careful guidance of the talented folks at the American Diabetes Association, and the collective wisdom of my colleagues and patients. I thank you all.

INTRODUCTION

Like many of my patients (and probably like you too), I sometimes feel like an overworked crazy person trying to get everything done. These are the times when it's especially important to remember—but easy to forget—both the desire and the obligation we have to take care of ourselves. The health-boosting strategies in this book will help you take care of yourself and your family in faster, better, and smarter ways. These are the strategies that have helped keep my patients and me sane and healthy. They can do the same for you.

Over the past two decades, I've counseled and coached thousands of patients. Some come to me in search of the magic weight loss plan—the one that will finally work (sadly, magic has nothing to do with it!); some people want to separate nutrition myth from fact (because there is a crazy lot of goofy stuff being tossed around as fact); and some simply want to learn how to make healthful eating fit with their busy lives. If you are in either of these latter two categories, *The Overworked Person's Guide to Better Nutrition* was written for you. Part 1 helps you organize your kitchen, offers strategies for faster meal preparation, and provides a blueprint for meal planning. If you feel that you're too busy or overworked right now to organize your kitchen and streamline your cooking, that's okay. Don't wait until you have more time to change your diet and start feeling healthier and more energetic. Get started today with Part 2. Come back to the first part of the book when you have more time.

After reading the introduction to Part 2, turn to any page for strategies to preserve nutrients in your food and to eat more disease-fighting nutrients and fewer disease-promoting foods. Learn to cut calories and slash sodium. You will find 50 practical ways to change your diet, live healthfully, and feel fabulous, even with your hectic life. *The Overworked Person's Guide to Better Nutrition* is not a weight loss program or a diet plan designed to control blood glucose, blood cholesterol, or any other health condition. But it is packed with tips to help you do all of these things. Some tips offer timesaving ideas; others are simple diet changes that cost you no time at all; and others are action plans that you can read and digest quickly to help you make smarter food and health decisions. You don't have to read an entire book to dive into better eating and health. In fact, if all you have is 5–10 free minutes, you will still be able to read a full health-boosting strategy and learn from it.

A lot of my patients know what to do—at least some of the time—but they don't know how to do it. RG was like that. He knew that he could lose weight and better control his diabetes if he ate more vegetables and fewer fast food sandwiches and highly processed snacks. He knew that he should exercise daily. But he didn't know how to squeeze exercise and balanced eating into his packed day. Like RG, you may know what to do but haven't had long-term success with weight loss, blood glucose control, keeping your energy up, cholesterol management, or other health and nutrition goals. That's because knowledge alone doesn't lead to behavior change. So if you know, for example, that eating more vegetables is good for you but you're still not eating them, this is the book to set you down a path of healthful eating.

A cautionary word here: Even though this book is written for people with hectic lives and gives you new information in a quick, easy-to-read format, implementing new strategies and forming new habits still take time. A timesaving strategy doesn't mean that you won't have to carve out any time at all. To make the best use of your limited time, work on the changes that are most important to you. Consistency is key, so pick a strategy and stick with it. That's what RG did, and now he's more than 50 pounds lighter and has his diabetes under better control.

Feel free to read the book from beginning to end, head straight to the topics most important to you, or simply open the book to a random page in Part 2 and get started. Or dig in deeper with the first two chapters to help you get organized and to speed up and simplify meal planning, preparation, and even cleanup. This is not an all-or-nothing guide. There are no rules here. Pick and choose what you like. If something in the book sounds like a good idea but you don't feel ready to make that change or it seems to be too difficult, give yourself permission to move on. Keep an open mind, and revisit the idea another day.

What can changing your diet do for you? Research tells us that a healthy diet and lifestyle can do quite a lot, such as:

- reduce your risk for type 2 diabetes, cardiovascular disease, dementia, bone loss, and several types of cancers

- control blood pressure, cholesterol, and glucose levels

- improve sleep quality

- slow cognitive decline among the elderly

- increase fertility

- heighten immune function

- aid in weight control

- help maintain focus on school or other tasks

- improve mood

- boost energy

- and so much more.

Get started, stay consistent, and you'll be victorious!

Disclosure Statement

In addition to working with patients, the author is a writer, speaker, consultant, and paid spokesperson. She works with certain brands and commodities because they fit with her nutrition philosophy, which promotes both healthfulness and great taste. No one has paid the author to mention or recommend any food or brand in this book. Each suggestion is based on the merits of the food. If you would like to see a list of the author's former and current clients, please visit jillweisenberger.com.

Part 1:

ORGANIZATION FOR YOU AND YOUR KITCHEN

Investing time in planning and organizing now frees up more time later. Carving out those initial minutes and hours is the hard part. If you don't have time right now to label shelves in your pantry or learn to plan meals, for example, skip over these first two chapters. You can still improve your diet and your health with each of the 50 strategies in the subsequent four chapters. Come back to Part 1 when the house is quiet and you're feeling motivated and energized to give your kitchen a health makeover.

Chapter 1:

THE ORGANIZED KITCHEN

This first chapter gets your kitchen in tip-top shape for healthful and more enjoyable cooking and eating. Stock up with the most nutritious, convenient, and versatile foods and the most practical utensils and appliances and arrange them in user-friendly ways.

Clear the Clutter

Clutter is a great distracter and time-waster. If you've ever been late for an appointment because you couldn't find the right clothes in an overstuffed closet, you know what I mean. If your refrigerator is home to rotting vegetables that you have forgotten were there, or if you open a second container of rice, oats, or walnuts because you can't find the first open container, then you could use a bit of organizing. If your kitchen counters or cabinets are full of small appliances and utensils that you never use, you will feel liberated by purging the waste. The time you put into organizing now will pay off many times over in time (and money) saved later.

1. SORT THROUGH YOUR STUFF.

Begin with just a couple of cabinets and drawers, or even just one. Line up five boxes, baskets, or bins, and identify them as follows: *Trash, Storage, Donate or Sell, Put Away–Kitchen*, and *Put Away–Elsewhere*. As you take things off the shelves and out of the drawers, put them in the appropriate containers. It may be hard to part with some things, especially if they were gifts or have sentimental value. Remind yourself that each extra dish, pot, and vegetable peeler gets in the way of quickly finding what you need. If you're struggling to label something as a keeper or a giveaway, put it in a sixth container. Label this one with a big question mark. Store the box with undecided items in the garage, attic, or elsewhere in the house. Come back to it in a few months or a year. If you haven't used an item in that time, it's probably safe to get rid of it.

Once you've emptied some space, take a few extra minutes to wipe down the shelves, doors, and drawers. If you like shelves lined with paper, this is the time to do it. Tackle your counters and every other space in the same manner. Remove everything, and put back only those things you need. If you have time to clear just one cabinet, that's okay. But if you can get through several cabinets, or the full kitchen, so much the better. Many people feel that they need big blocks of time to accomplish chores. Not so! If you take 30 minutes to clean out a small space, you will be 30 minutes closer to your goal. But if you wait until you have a couple of free hours, then that unused half hour was wasted. The same principle applies to not exercising because you're crunched for time. Half of your usual walk is better than no walk, and one organized cabinet is better than no organized cabinets.

2. BE SMART WITH STORAGE.

In the process of cleaning and organizing your kitchen, make a designated place for everything. You'll be able to cook and clean much faster if things are not scattered about or missing. I know. I've burned many a dish while fishing through drawers for tongs or a spatula.

- Tuck away anything you don't use on a regular basis. If you rarely drink coffee, there's no need to leave your coffeemaker on the counter just because that's where it's always been. If you use it daily, however, making a home for it near both your sink and an electrical outlet makes good sense.

- Corral like items. Keep all of your measuring cups and spoons in one place, so you're not hunting around the kitchen looking for just the right one. Fill an attractive canister or jar with everyday cooking utensils such as mixing spoons, spatulas, and tongs. Keep them near your stove where you will need them.

- Consider buying drawer organizers for your kitchen tools.

- Hang your potholders near the oven so they're easy to grab, but not so close that they're a fire hazard.

- If you reuse plastic grocery bags, mount a bag holder on the inside of a cabinet door. You can find one for about $10 in kitchen shops.

- Don't be a prisoner to your current shelving arrangement. If your shelves are removable, move them around to fit your needs. Get creative if you need additional space. You can find vinyl-coated wire organizer shelves in most home-improvement and kitchen stores. I have several, allowing me to stack things that otherwise wouldn't be stackable. If you need vertical space for platters, roasting pans, or cookie sheets, purchase vertical racks to fit inside your cabinet. Or make your own vertical dividers with tension curtain rods (used to hang curtains). Buy several rods to fit between two shelves, and line them up an inch or two apart, or whatever distance fits your cutting boards, platters, etc.

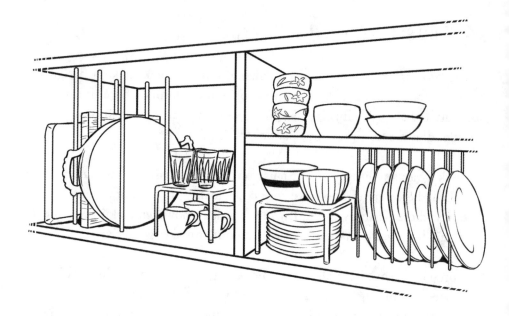

✌ Use a lazy Susan or turntable to store small items such as spice bottles, teabags, or sweeteners. I have my spices on a two-tier lazy Susan that I spin quickly to find whatever spice I've just decided my dish must have. I even have my seasonings organized alphabetically. Before I took the time to alphabetize them, I had several duplicate open bottles. Inevitably, I couldn't find my open paprika, cinnamon, or rosemary, so I'd assume that I had run out. Eventually, I'd find two open bottles of the same thing.

✌ Add hanging racks or baskets to the inside of your cabinet doors. Use them for cleaning supplies or for small items such as measuring cups or spoons.

3. USE THE SAME PRINCIPLES IN YOUR PANTRY, REFRIGERATOR, AND FREEZER.

✌ Corral like items.

- A turntable isn't just for your kitchen cabinets. Use one in the refrigerator for the condiments and small bottles that don't fit in the door.

- Gather all of your sandwich-making foods in an open basket, so that when it's time to pack lunch, you can simply grab the container out of the refrigerator and quickly put a sandwich together.

- Arrange things in your pantry to prevent having multiple open packages of the same item. Either store the opened and unopened rice together and the opened and unopened lentils together, or keep all of the opened packages in one bin and all of the unopened packages in a separate bin.

✌ Organize your pantry so that it makes sense to you. If you have lots of small items, it might be better to line your shelves with containers to store most of your pantry items. Or you can purchase tiered shelf organizers to stack cans, bottles, and other items. Stack baking items like flour and sugar in plastic or glass storage containers. Similarly, arrange your refrigerator and freezer in ways that work for you and your family.

- Follow FIFO—First In, First Out. When putting packaged soups in your pantry or yogurt in your refrigerator, store them in such a way that you use the oldest item first.

- Now that you have an organized pantry, refrigerator, and freezer, label your shelves, storage containers, and turntables, so that everyone in your household knows where to store new groceries or return whatever food they just took out.

4. KNOW WHAT YOU HAVE.

- Old cottage cheese or margarine containers have no place in a busy cook's kitchen. Invest in glass or good plastic see-through containers for the refrigerator and pantry, so you can easily tell what's inside them.

- As soon as you open a carton of chicken stock, a jar of pasta sauce, or a container of hummus, write the date on it with a thick marker. Next time you reach for it, check the date to be certain it's still fresh. Remind family members to do the same. Remind them often, if necessary. I can't count the number of times I've found opened but unmarked pasta sauce jars in my refrigerator.

- Keep a grocery list close at hand, and add to it every time you open the last box of shredded wheat, jar of mustard, or any staple item in your home. If you go through canned tomatoes quickly, for example, add them to your list before you get to the last can. If you think you might stop by the grocery store but you don't want to remove the list from the kitchen, snap a picture of it with your smartphone. If you do find time to run into the market, you'll have your list handy. (Some people prefer to keep a running list in their smartphones.) To save time, organize your shopping list so that it follows the floor plan of your supermarket. See the appendix for a grocery list template, and modify it so that it fits your needs. Another option is a supermarket app. Here are a few to consider:

- Grocery IQ (groceryiq.com) allows you to sort your list by aisle; app has barcode scanning.

- Ziplist (get.ziplist.com) allows you to put recipes from the web into your recipe box and enter the ingredients into your shopping list; app has barcode scanning.

- Out of Milk (outofmilk.com) allows you to make multiple lists and allows for adding details such as price, quantity, and coupons; app includes a Pantry List for you to keep track of each item currently in your pantry.

Timesaving Tools

There are so many very cool kitchen appliances and tools out there. Below is a list of kitchen items that are timesavers for many people. Before investing in anything else that can add to the clutter, however, really think about how you will use these tools and if they will be timesavers for you or simply space-grabbers.

RICE COOKER: It may seem silly to purchase an appliance to cook just rice, but you'll be surprised at just how versatile a rice cooker is. You can use it to prepare most grains, including quinoa, barley, farro, wheat berries, and even oats. Most rice cookers allow you to steam vegetables as well. The main reason I love my rice cooker is that I can turn it on and walk away. There's no waiting for liquid to boil and then lowering the temperature. I don't have to set the timer or come back to make sure that what I'm cooking doesn't burn. The appliance cooks the grain and turns itself off automatically. It even keeps the food warm. My rice cooker is a true timesaver for me.

FOOD PROCESSOR: If you do lots of slicing, dicing, shredding, and grating, a food processor is a smart purchase and will save you time. It's easy to bulk up portions of lasagna, casseroles, pasta salads, spaghetti sauce, tuna salad, and more dishes if you have sliced and diced veggies on the ready. If space is tight or if you want to keep the cost down, buy a mini food processor.

INDUSTRIAL-STRENGTH BLENDER: This is an expensive appliance but worth every penny if you use it often to consume some of nature's most nutritious foods—fruits and vegetables. I use a Vitamix. Blendtec and Breville are similar brands. Because these blenders are so powerful, you don't need to finely chop each ingredient or use and wash several appliances and pots to prepare a single recipe. Process almonds to make almond butter or almond milk. Toss in the fruits and vegetables you have on hand for a smoothie or blended juice drink. A few salad vegetables, tomato juice, and seasoning will give you gazpacho, a delicious summery cold soup. Or if you prefer a hot soup, add your ingredients and process for several minutes until it's piping hot.

IMMERSION BLENDER: Also called a stick blender, an immersion blender lets you blend or purée right in the cooking pot. Using one is easier, faster, and safer than transferring hot liquids between the pot and a traditional stand blender. It's quick to wash as well. Use it for puréed soups and to purée cooked vegetables to add to casseroles, meatloaf, and many other dishes.

PRESSURE COOKER: This appliance cooks food in a fraction of the time that a traditional pot on the stove would take. Beans are done in minutes instead of hours. You can prepare a pot roast in 30–45 minutes and artichokes in less than 10 minutes. The hitch is that the preparation time is no shorter. If lengthy cooking times slow you down, a pressure cooker may be a smart buy. But if you're looking to save time with the prep and cleanup, this isn't the appliance to help you.

SLOW COOKER: It sounds odd that you can save time with something called a slow cooker. But this is another one of those fix-it-and-walk-away appliances. To get the most out of your slow cooker, you'll need to plan your menu in advance to have all of your ingredients on hand. To avoid the morning rush, chop vegetables and measure herbs the night before. In the morning, take the ingredients out of the refrigerator and place them all in the slow cooker insert. Turn it on, and off you go. Use a slow cooker liner for super-fast cleanup. If you have sports practices, late meetings at the office, or some other activity that brings you home late, the slow cooker is a great way to have a healthful, home-cooked dinner ready when you are. When my kids had soccer, gymnastics, and field hockey night after night, I had my slow cooker in regular use.

✌ Getting Started Tips

To prevent washed-out flavors in your slow cooker, use more seasonings than usual and plenty of aromatics like garlic and onions. To prevent overcooked, mushy vegetables, add spinach, zucchini, and other tender vegetables in the last 20 or 30 minutes. Another way to avoid overcooking vegetables is to toss carrots, fennel, potatoes, and other favorite vegetables in a bit of oil and seasonings, wrap them in a foil packet, and place the packet on top of the other ingredients.

PANINI PRESS: I love a Panini press to make a quick yet fancy sandwich for lunch or dinner. What could be better and faster than throwing some favorite ingredients between two slices of bread and then between the grill plates of a Panini press? Like a rice cooker, a Panini press sounds limited in function. But also like a rice cooker, it's a multitasker. Instead of heating your big outdoor grill, use your Panini press to cook whatever you would cook outside. Finish dinner with grilled fruit such as peaches, figs, or pineapple. Just slice, toss onto the grill plate, and close.

SALAD SPINNER: A salad spinner dries lettuce, spinach, other vegetables, and even fruits better than other methods. I sometimes use mine to dry frozen vegetables after I've defrosted them and before using them in recipes.

VEGETABLE PEELER: It's much faster to skin an apple or potato with a vegetable peeler, preferably one with a swivel blade, than with a knife. Typically, a vegetable peeler removes less of the flesh too. Use it also to slice chocolate curls and thin pieces of cheese.

HAND JUICER: A tablespoon or two of citrus juice goes a long way to flavor a dish, especially when you are trimming sodium. A hand juicer does a great job of giving you the juice without the seeds—plus it's quick to use and wash.

DIGITAL SCALE: Rather than using a measuring cup to measure a serving of cottage cheese or other food, then transferring it to the bowl you're going to eat from, you can put the bowl on the scale; you save time and a transfer. You also have one less thing to wash.

NONSTICK BAKING MAT: I used to think that this was an expensive luxury. Not anymore! A baking mat makes for super-fast and easy cleanup. Line any baking sheet or pan with it, and you'll have the dishes washed in seconds. Use it for roasting vegetables, baking fish or chicken, and even making cookies. It's better than lining your pan with aluminum foil because you don't have the waste.

KITCHEN SHEARS: Cut everything from herbs to pizza to chicken parts. It's much less work than using a knife.

❧ Do It Fast Tips

Buy a pair of kitchen shears that comes apart for quick, easy washing.

OTHER FAVORITE TOOLS: Having useful tools for healthful cooking allows you to do more in less time. I use each of the following on a regular basis: microwave, oil mister, heat-resistant spatulas and spoons, tongs, measuring spoons and measuring cups, vegetable steamer, colanders, cutting boards, digital timer, digital thermometer, sharp knives, and a knife sharpener.

Stock Your Kitchen with Good-for-You Foods

None of those utensils and appliances will do you a bit of good if you don't have the right groceries handy. This list will get you started.

Pantry

In general, it's best to purchase packaged goods with little or no added sugars and salt.

CANNED TOMATOES: I love these for their versatility. They punch up pasta, soups, and casseroles, and they're terrific with fish, chicken, refried beans, and black beans.

PASTA SAUCE: Compare brands for sodium, saturated fat, and added sugars.

SALSA: Yes, it counts as a vegetable! Add it to cold pasta for a fast salad, pour it over chicken or fish before baking, or mix it with nonfat Greek yogurt for a nutritious 10-second veggie dip.

CANNED BEANS AND FAT-FREE REFRIED BEANS: Use these to put a meatless meal on the table very quickly.

DRIED LENTILS: Lentils, especially red lentils, are the fastest legume to cook. Make a quick soup, salad, or side dish.

CANNED OR POUCHED TUNA AND SALMON: Make a nutritious sandwich or a simple salad lickety-split.

REDUCED-SODIUM BROTH: Cooking with broth is a smart way to cut back on salt and fat. Simmer rice, quinoa, and other whole grains in broth instead of salted water with butter. Be sure to compare labels for fat as well as sodium.

CANNED SOUPS: Look for a low-sodium variety. Soups like black bean and lentil make the better part of a meal.

MARINATED ARTICHOKE HEARTS: Shake off the extra oil and toss these into a green salad. They are so flavorful that you can omit or reduce the salad dressing. Brighten up tuna salad, flatbreads, omelets, and all kinds of things.

SUN-DRIED TOMATOES: These also liven up a variety of foods, including fish, chicken, and pasta salads. Use either the plain or marinated kind. (Again, I prefer marinated for their flavor.) To keep the calories down, drain the oil and reduce the amount of additional oil or dressing in your recipe.

WHOLE GRAINS: This category includes whole-wheat pasta, brown rice, wild rice, wheat berries, farro, barley, and quinoa. Have instant and quick-cooking varieties on hand for a speedy side dish.

WHOLE-GRAIN BREAD PRODUCTS: Choose flatbread, sandwich bread, pita, English muffins, bagel thins, crackers, tortillas, or any favorite. For portion control, choose bagel thins, small corn or flour tortillas, mini pita breads, and thinly sliced breads. Unless you go through it quickly, it's smart to keep whole-grain bread in the freezer and defrost just a slice or two as needed.

CANNED FRUIT: With this in the pantry, there's no excuse to have a meal without fruit. Look for the no-sugar-added varieties.

TOMATO OR VEGETABLE JUICE: These juices are perfect for taking the edge off your hunger before a meal. An 8-ounce serving has only about 50 calories and 10 grams of carbohydrate. The low-sodium variety is ideal.

NUTS: Add crunch to salads and whole grain pilafs, or enjoy a handful for a snack. Limit your portion to about an ounce (about 1/4 cup) because nuts are heavy on calories. Fortunately, most of the fat they have is the good-for-you kind.

NUT BUTTERS: Peanut butter, almond butter, and others make a great quick breakfast, lunch, or snack when spread on whole-grain bread or tart apple slices.

CANOLA AND OLIVE OILS: Both contain the healthy omega-9 monounsaturated fats, and canola oil is a good source of omega-3 fatty acids.

VINEGARS: Add a healthy pizzazz to everything from chicken to cooked or raw leafy greens to black beans with vinegars like balsamic, sherry, and cider. I admit to being a balsamic nut and drizzle it on salads, salmon, beef, onions, and even grilled figs and peaches.

TEA: Keep a few varieties on hand to enjoy hot or cold.

HERBS AND SPICES: Purchase the ones you use frequently in medium or large jars. For those you use only rarely, buy as little as a spoonful from a store that sells them in bulk. Save empty jars to store your bulk seasonings. If you prefer spice blends, read the labels carefully and buy the sodium-free varieties.

Refrigerator and Freezer

NONFAT PLAIN GREEK YOGURT: This is an ingredient that has many more uses than first appears. Mix it with fresh or frozen fruit for a nutrient-packed breakfast or snack, turn it into a smoothie, and stir it into sauces for added creaminess. Use it instead of sour cream or mayonnaise in dressings.

STRONG CHEESES LIKE PARMESAN, FETA, BLUE, AND SHARP CHEDDAR: Since these are so pungent, you don't need to use much for a flavor boost. A sprinkling of feta cheese over whole grains or grated Parmesan over chicken or vegetables adds flavor and complexity.

LOW-FAT COTTAGE CHEESE: For a protein boost at breakfast, I mix cottage cheese with cinnamon and raisins, spread it on toasted whole-grain raisin bread (I like the Food for Life brand), and pop it in the toaster oven until warm and fragrant. Try cottage cheese with tomatoes and basil for a low-carb snack, or mix it with your favorite berries for a sweet treat. I like Daisy Brand 2% Cottage Cheese because of its simple ingredients list; it has no food starches or anything else that adds carbohydrate and dilutes the protein.

HUMMUS: It's a ready-made dip for veggies or whole-grain pita bread.

FRESH AND FROZEN VEGETABLES: Fill half your plate with nonstarchy vegetables such as cauliflower, carrots, tomatoes, zucchini, and broccoli. Save yourself a few trips to the grocery store by stocking up on frozen vegetables. See the box on page 21 for a list of nonstarchy vegetables.

EDAMAME BEANS: Purchase these in the pod or shelled. They cook up quickly in boiling water. Eat them with just a sprinkling of salt right from the pod, or add the shelled beans to salads and whole-grain pilafs. Edamame beans are high in both fiber and protein. In fact, half of the carbohydrate comes from fiber, making them an especially good snack or addition to a meal.

READY-TO-EAT BEETS: This food is the ultimate in convenience. Just open the refrigerated package—Love Beets, Melissa's Produce, and Trader Joe's are a few available brands—and add delicious, nutritious beets to your salad. *Hint:* For a fun salad, dice a couple of beets and toss with a chopped scallion and walnuts. Top with a dollop of nonfat plain Greek yogurt.

BAGGED SALAD GREENS, LETTUCE, OR BABY SPINACH: What could be a faster start to a health-boosting salad?

FRESH AND FROZEN FRUIT: Don't be worried that fruit is bad for your blood glucose. If you have diabetes, just count the carbohydrate in fruit as you would with any food. You can learn more about carbohydrate counting here: http://www.diabetes.org/food-and-fitness/food/what-can-i-eat/understanding-carbohydrates/carbohydrate-counting.html. Or ask your physician for a referral to a registered dietitian nutritionist (RD or RDN).

LIMES AND LEMONS: Brighten up the flavor of whole grains, vegetables, salads, fish, and poultry with grated peel or a squeeze of citrus.

BOTTLED GINGER: If you like ginger, you'll love the taste and ease of bottled ginger. The Spice World brand can often be found in the supermarket produce section. It's almost as delicious as freshly grated ginger but much more convenient.

GROUND MEAT: Select 90% lean or leaner for quick meals like tortilla soup, taco salads, and spaghetti sauce. Don't be duped by the health halo of ground turkey. It might be ground with skin, so read the label.

FROZEN EASY-PEEL SHRIMP: Defrost it quickly under running water. Then sauté or stir-fry with your favorite veggies for a fast, easy meal.

FRESH AND FROZEN FISH: Choose salmon, tuna, trout, and herring for their omega-3 fatty acids.

FRESH AND FROZEN CHICKEN: To save time (and unhealthy saturated fats), buy it skinless or remove the skin after purchasing and rewrap the meat. Frozen chicken pieces defrost quickly in a bowl of cold water. I especially like chicken tenderloins because they're so fast to cook. They're good for baking, sautéing, or stir-frying after dicing.

EGGS OR EGG SUBSTITUTE: Eggs are perhaps the fastest protein food to cook, and they work well for all three meals—plus they're an inexpensive protein source. Because egg yolks are high in dietary cholesterol, limit the yolks and use more whites than yolks.

FROZEN MEALS: These are better than most fast food choices for the times you're running late or when you simply need a break from cooking. Both frozen and shelf-stable meals should have:

- no more than 500 calories (about 350 calories for weight loss)

- no more than 3 grams saturated fat

- 0 grams trans fat

- no more than 600 mg sodium, but preferably less than 480 mg

- carbohydrate to match your meal plan if you have diabetes

- at least 3 grams fiber, but preferably 5 grams or more

- at least 14 grams protein.

Add a serving of something nutritious to round out your meal. For example, add a salad to boost your veggie intake, a glass of milk to get more protein and calcium, or a piece of fruit to ring up more fiber.

Here are a few frozen meals to try. Since manufacturers periodically change their recipes, review the Nutrition Facts panel before purchase. If you have diabetes, pay close attention to the amount of carbohydrate in each frozen meal.

- Lean Cuisine Beef Chow Fun

- Lean Cuisine Salad Additions™ Asian-Style Chicken Salad

- Lean Cuisine Salad Additions™ Southwestern-Style Chicken Salad

- Healthy Choice Grilled Chicken Pesto with Vegetables

- Healthy Choice Herb Crusted Fish

- Kashi® Chicken Pasta Pomodoro

- Weight Watchers Smart Ones Home Style Beef Pot Roast

Nonstarchy Vegetables

You should put vegetables of all types on your menu for a bevy of health-boosting nutrients and delicious flavor. Nonstarchy varieties, however, are lower in calories and carbohydrates, making them perfect choices for weight watchers and anyone with diabetes. Aim for a couple of cups each day. Think beyond green beans and broccoli. Here is just a partial list.

Artichokes and artichoke hearts	Cucumbers	Salad greens and leaves, including arugula, chicory, endive, lettuce, radicchio, and watercress
Asparagus	Eggplant	Sprouts, such as alfalfa, bean, broccoli, and soybean (see Health-Boosting Strategy #37 on page 108 for a safety warning)
Bamboo shoots	Greens, such as collards, kale, mustard, and turnip	Squashes, such as crookneck, pattypan, yellow, and zucchini
Beets	Hearts of palm	Sugar snap peas
Broccoli	Jicama	Swiss chard
Broccoli rabe (also called rapini)	Kohlrabi	Tomato juice
Brussels sprouts	Mushrooms	Tomatoes
Cabbages, such as green, purple, bok choy, and Chinese	Okra	Turnips
Carrots	Onions, including sweet, yellow, purple, scallions, shallots, and leeks	Vegetable juice, preferably reduced- or low-sodium
Cauliflower	Peppers, including bell and spicy	Water chestnuts
Celery		

Hungry for more information about vegetables and ways to cook them? Visit Fruits and Veggies More Matters® (fruitsandveggiesmorematters.org).

Chapter 2:

THE ORGANIZED MENU

Meal planning is challenging, but a healthful diet requires some level of planning. The rewards include saving money, meeting nutritional goals, and avoiding what I call the dinner frenzy—that mad race to pull dinner together with no plan and no time. Sometimes even the best planners haven't made developing basic meal-planning skills a priority. Fortunately, they are simple skills that everyone can learn and turn into a habit. In this chapter, you'll learn various methods of meal planning and find several ways to put a healthful meal on the table faster and better than ever before.

Meal Planning

There are several ways to plan meals. I follow a very flexible, unstructured meal-planning process that gives me a general idea of the food I will prepare for my family for the coming week. This is a quick method. Many of my patients also prefer it, but some like a more formal, structured process. Both are described here.

Mix-and-Match Meal Planning

There are four simple steps to this flexible method.

1. LOOK AHEAD.

No matter how tempting it is, don't skip this critical step. Ask yourself what obstacles may prevent you from getting a planned dinner on the table. Do you have a late meeting this week, or will you be driving your kids to soccer practice one or two evenings? Is this your week to volunteer at the food bank? If you answer yes, pick a meal that can be prepared in advance, or use one of the Recipes on the Ready ideas in this chapter. Use the template in the Appendix to organize your selections.

2. SELECT ENTRÉES AND SIDE DISHES.

If, for example, you need to plan five dinners, choose five main courses, five starches, and five nonstarchy vegetables. You do not need to plan the full meal, but do be certain to list enough choices in each category to make the necessary number of full meals. For example, you might plan to prepare baked salmon, roasted chicken, black beans and rice, spaghetti with meat sauce, and oven-fried tilapia. You'll need three starches for the meals that don't already include pasta or rice, five nonstarchy vegetables, and salad vegetables for most or all of the evenings. As long as you have these foods on hand, you don't need to decide which night you'll prepare each item, or even which side dishes to match with the entrées.

3. TAKE INVENTORY.

Now that you've selected the foods and recipes to prepare, identify which ingredients you have on hand. Add to your grocery list anything you don't have. Don't feel compelled to preselect which vegetables and other side dishes to buy. As long as you know the proper number, you can decide in the supermarket. Make your selections based on what looks good and what is affordable.

4. FILL IN THE REST OF THE MEALS.

In a similar manner, consider your lunches. Do you pack lunch, eat lunch at home, or do you alternate? Select the required number of fruits, vegetables, sandwich meats, etc. Add the necessary items to your list. Do the same for the foods you will need for breakfasts and snacks.

Detailed Meal Planning

This process follows the same basic principles, but you make your decisions and your plan in more detail.

1. LOOK AHEAD.

Just as in the mix-and-match meal-planning process, look at your calendar and find out from others about any upcoming obstacles to an easy family dinner or a relaxing dinner for one.

2. PUT YOUR PLAN ON PAPER.

Using any type of calendar or the template in the Appendix, jot down full dinners that you plan to prepare. Typically plan a meat or vegetarian entrée, a starchy food, and one or more nonstarchy vegetables. Fruit for dessert or with the meal is also a good idea. You can start with the most hectic days and pick meals from the Recipes on the Ready section, or you can begin with your most flexible days, planning leftovers for the busier evenings. For example, you might plan to serve steak, small baked potatoes, green beans, and salad on Tuesday when you can be home early. Because your Wednesday is more hectic, you can use leftover steak in a steak sandwich, and serve it with leftover salad.

If you have been using the Plate Method to guide your food choices, you can continue to do so. There is a template in the Appendix for structured meal planning using the Plate Method. With this method, you draw an imaginary line down the center of your 9-inch dinner plate. Fill one half of the plate with nonstarchy vegetables, and divide the other half between approximately equal portions of a starchy food (such as potatoes or rice) and a protein-rich food (such as fish or chicken). To learn more about the Plate Method or to get a refresher, visit the website of the American Diabetes Association (http://www.diabetes.org/food-and-fitness/food/planning-meals/create-your-plate).

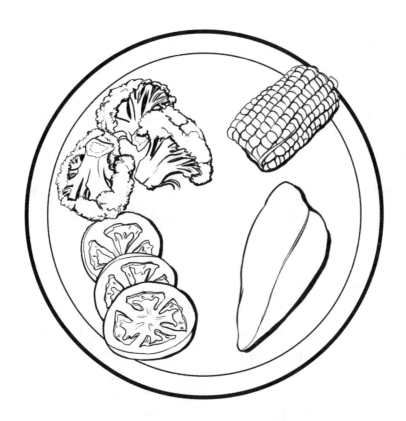

If you're new to meal planning, make it easy on yourself and start with your favorite meals. You probably have a dozen or at least half a dozen favorite meals. Fill in your calendar with some of those meals first; then add the rest of the evening meals. Be sure to match the complexity of the meal with the amount of time you have available for preparation. If you'd like, continue with this process for lunches and breakfasts. If you're comfortable with your current plan for lunches and breakfasts, then just focus on dinner. Remember, part of making the best use of your time and your energy is narrowing your focus to what matters most.

3. TAKE INVENTORY.

Add to your grocery list any ingredients or staple items that you don't have on hand.

4. BUILD FLEXIBILITY INTO YOUR PLAN.

If an item is on special at the grocery store or if you simply have a desire to try something new, go for it. A plan is your guide, not a set of rules that you must follow. Make it work for you by remaining flexible. Let's say you plan to cook chicken tonight, but something keeps you from getting home on time—or better yet, you have reason to celebrate and choose to eat out. Simply wrap the chicken tightly and toss it in the freezer or switch plans to cook it tomorrow. Enjoy your night out, or prepare a quick dinner with other foods you have on hand.

5. RECYCLE YOUR MENUS.

Make everything as easy on yourself as possible. (This one directive is critical to the success of meal planning and everything else described in this book. If a strategy is too difficult, you won't be able to stick with it for long.) Without allowing yourself to get into a food rut, reuse what works. Keep your menus in a paper folder or on your computer. After you have three or four weeks of menus, take the best from each week's menu to create the next week's.

Get Comfortable in the Kitchen

If you don't have basic cooking skills, it's worth developing them. The more competent you are in the kitchen, the more quickly you can get a meal on the table. You will save time by improvising, substituting, and estimating, and by relying less on recipes. Another bonus is that cooking puts you in control of what you eat, so you can eat better. It's easier to estimate calories for weight control and carbohydrates for blood glucose control when you know the ingredients in your meals. You can trim calories, saturated fats, sodium, and carbohydrates when you wear the chef's hat.

If you have time and it interests you, take a cooking class at your local college or community center. If you'd rather teach yourself, look for either of my two favorite resources:

❧ *How to Cook Everything* by Mark Bittman, book and iPhone app

❧ *Cooking Light Way to Cook: The Complete Visual Guide to Everyday Cooking*

Faster, Better, Smarter Cooking Techniques

You probably rarely, if ever, have the luxury of leisurely preparing a big meal with a dozen or more major ingredients and as many pots, pans, and utensils to clean up afterward. And even if you do, you'd probably want to spend the time somewhere other than the kitchen! By becoming a master of a few smart cooking techniques, you can reap the rewards of nutritious, tasty, home-prepared meals and avoid being a slave to your oven or stove. Start with the following two super-fast, super-easy cooking methods.

Parchment Paper Cooking—Dinner Is All Wrapped Up

With this cooking technique, the designated dishwasher in your house will become your biggest fan. There are no pots and little mess. Cleanup is as simple as tossing a few things in the dishwasher, rinsing off a baking sheet, and throwing used parchment paper in the trash. Absolutely nothing more! My husband, the cleanup guy in our house, is the biggest devotee of parchment paper cooking I know. He's out of the kitchen in less than 10 minutes.

You can prepare an entrée, side dish, or entire meal in parchment paper. I prefer to create the whole meal in a packet. Below are four recipes that are popular in my house. You can use them exactly as written, but it's even better to follow them as a guide to create your own recipes, or modify your favorite recipes to fit this simple five-step formula.

1. Cut a 20-inch piece of parchment paper. Fold it in half and open it back up. *Hint:* The parchment paper stays open better if you fold it in the direction opposite to its natural curve.

2. Scoop cooked and chilled grains such as brown rice, farro, wheat berries, or spaghetti onto the parchment paper. Center the food on only one side of the fold. Flatten the mound of food so the thickness is fairly even throughout.

3. Top the grain with a vegetable and a protein-rich food like shrimp or chicken. Season with herbs, spices, olive oil, or a sauce, as appropriate.

4. Fold the parchment paper so the meal is within the packet, and wrap tightly on each of the three sides (see the diagram below).

5. Place the packet on a cookie sheet and bake until the meat has come to a safe internal temperature and the vegetables are tender. See Health-Boosting Strategy #38 on page 110 for safe minimum temperatures.

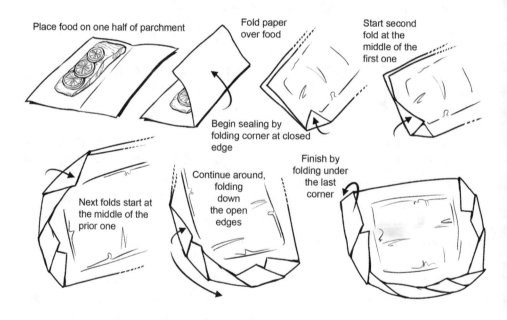

Double, triple, or halve each recipe depending on the number of people at your table. I often make an extra packet so that I can have a meal ready for my lunch the following day. Occasionally, to save even more time, I make one large packet with aluminum foil instead of several smaller packets with parchment paper. You will find more parchment paper recipes on the Internet and in the book *The Parchment Paper Cookbook* by Brette Sember.

Southwestern Chicken and Rice

1	cup prepared brown rice
1/4	cup no-salt-added canned kidney beans, drained and rinsed
8	ounces of chicken tenderloins (or other chicken breast that is not very thick)
1/4	teaspoon black pepper
1/8	teaspoon ground cumin
1/4	teaspoon garlic powder
1/4	cup salsa
6	small black olives, sliced
2	tablespoons shredded reduced-fat sharp Cheddar cheese

1. Preheat oven to 400°F. Cut two 20-inch pieces of parchment paper.

2. Place 1/2 cup rice and 2 tablespoons beans on each piece of parchment paper. Top with chicken. Spread seasonings, salsa, and olives evenly over chicken.

3. Fold parchment tightly so that none of the juices will leak out. Place packets on a baking sheet. Bake for 18 minutes or until chicken is cooked through. Carefully open each packet and sprinkle 1 tablespoon cheese over chicken.

Yield: 2 packets. Serves: 2. Serving Size: 1 packet.
Exchanges/Choices: 2 Starch, 1/2 Vegetable, 3 Lean Meat, 1/4 Medium-Fat Meat
Calories: 303
Total Fat: 6g/ Saturated Fat: 2g/ Trans Fat: 0g/ Cholesterol: 78mg/ Sodium: 518mg/
Total Carbohydrate: 30g/ Dietary Fiber: 5g/ Sugars: 2g/ Protein: 30g

Tarragon Chicken with Potatoes

2   tablespoons light mayonnaise

1 1/2 teaspoons Dijon mustard

1   tablespoon chopped tarragon

2   small potatoes, about 5 ounces each, sliced 1/8 inch thick

8   ounces of chicken tenderloins (or other chicken breast that is not very thick)

1/8   teaspoon kosher or other coarse salt

1/8   teaspoon black pepper

1/8   teaspoon garlic powder

6   medium mushrooms, sliced (about 4 ounces)

1. Preheat oven to 400°F. Cut two 20-inch pieces of parchment paper.

2. Mix light mayonnaise, Dijon mustard, and chopped tarragon together. Set aside.

3. Place half the sliced potatoes on each piece of parchment paper. Dot with half the sauce and spread over potatoes. Top with chicken. Spread remaining sauce over chicken.

4. Sprinkle chicken with salt, pepper, and garlic powder. Put sliced mushrooms around the chicken.

5. Fold parchment tightly so that none of the juices leak out. Place packets on a baking sheet. Bake for 17–20 minutes or until chicken is cooked through.

Yield: 2 packets. Serves: 2. Serving Size: 1 packet.
Exchanges/Choices: 1/2 Vegetable, 3 Lean Meat, 1 Fat, 1 Starch
Calories: 309
Total Fat: 8g/ Saturated Fat: 1.5g/ Trans Fat: 0g/ Cholesterol: 78mg/ Sodium: 445mg/
Total Carbohydrate: 29g/ Dietary Fiber: 3g/ Sugars: 2g/ Protein: 28g

Garlic Shrimp over Spaghetti and Asparagus

2	tablespoons olive oil
1	teaspoon sodium-free lemon pepper
1/4	teaspoon kosher or other coarse salt
1/4	teaspoon black pepper, preferably coarse ground
2	garlic cloves, chopped
1	pound shrimp, shells and tails removed
2 2/3	cups cooked whole-grain spaghetti
16	asparagus spears, cut into 2-inch pieces

1. Preheat oven to 400°F. Cut four 20-inch pieces of parchment paper.

2. Mix together olive oil, lemon pepper, salt, pepper, and garlic. Pour over shrimp and mix.

3. Place 2/3 cup spaghetti on each piece of parchment paper. Top with one quarter of the asparagus and one quarter of the seasoned shrimp.

4. Fold parchment tightly so that none of the juices leak out. Place packets on a baking sheet. Bake for 12–14 minutes or until shrimp is opaque and pearly and asparagus is tender.

Yield: 4 packets, each with about 7–8 large shrimp. Serves: 4. Serving Size: 1 packet.
Exchanges/Choices: 1/2 Vegetable, 2 1/2 Lean Meat, 1 1/2 Fat, 2 Starch
Calories: 263
Total Fat: 8g/ Saturated Fat: 1g/ Trans Fat: 0g/ Cholesterol: 135mg/ Sodium: 211mg/
Total Carbohydrate: 28g/ Dietary Fiber: 5g/ Sugars: 2g/ Protein: 24g

Salmon and Quinoa with Broccoli

1	cup cooked quinoa
2	skinless salmon fillets, 4 ounces each
2	cups broccoli florets, large pieces (about 4 ounces)
8	cherry tomatoes
1/8	teaspoon salt
1/8	teaspoon pepper
1/8	teaspoon garlic powder
1/8	teaspoon dried dill weed or 1/4–1/2 teaspoon fresh, chopped dill weed

Squeeze of fresh lemon or 1/2–1 teaspoon lemon juice

1. Preheat oven to 400°F. Cut two 20-inch pieces of parchment paper.

2. Place 1/2 cup quinoa on each piece of parchment paper. Top with 4 ounces salmon. Spread 1 cup broccoli florets and 4 cherry tomatoes around salmon. Sprinkle with salt, pepper, garlic powder, and dill. Squeeze fresh lemon or drizzle bottled lemon juice over the entire mound of food.

3. Fold parchment tightly. Place packets on a baking sheet. Bake for 16–18 minutes or until salmon is cooked through and broccoli is tender.

Yield: 2 packets. Serves: 2. Serving Size: 1 packet.
Exchanges/Choices: 1 Vegetable, 3 Medium-Fat Meat, 1 1/2 Starch
Calories: 381
Total Fat: 17g/ Saturated Fat: 4g/ Trans Fat: 0g/ Cholesterol: 62mg/ Sodium: 242mg/
Total Carbohydrate: 27g/ Dietary Fiber: 6g/ Sugars: 3g/ Protein: 30g

Stir-Fry Meals in Minutes

If you have everything prepped earlier in the day, you can have dinner on the table within 15 minutes of walking into the kitchen. What goes into your wok or pan is limited only by your creativity. To keep your meals interesting, think beyond Asian seasonings. There's no reason that soy sauce has to be featured in every stir-fry dish. In fact, sauces of any kind are optional. Below are some steps to stir-fry success and two recipes to show you just how simple it is.

1. Because you'll move quickly, it's critical to have *all* of your ingredients ready to go—chopped, sliced, and measured—before turning on the heat. If you have time, cut and gather all of your ingredients earlier in the day, or even the day before. To save even more time, buy precut vegetables in your supermarket produce section, or choose frozen vegetables. Use either leftover rice or another grain, or start cooking it early. If you're having fruit or salad, be sure that too is ready to serve.

2. Slice beef, poultry, or pork thinly for fast cooking. Partially freeze for easier cutting. For another timesaver, ask the butcher in the grocery store to preslice your meat. Buy extra, and freeze it for another time.

3. Heat the pan before adding the oil, and heat the oil before adding the meats or vegetables.

4. Be sure that your vegetables are dry before adding them to the pan.

5. If cooking all of the vegetables at once, cut quick-cooking ones like mushrooms in large pieces and longer-cooking vegetables like broccoli in smaller pieces. Or cut them evenly and add them to the pan according to their cooking time, with the firmest vegetables going in first.

6. Stir-fry in batches. Overcrowding the pan adds excess moisture and steams your food instead of stir-frying it.

7. Add the sauce when the food is largely cooked. I rarely thicken soy sauce or other sauce with cornstarch. Feel free to take the extra step, though, if you prefer a thicker sauce.

8. If not using a sauce, keep a spoonful of water or low-sodium broth nearby. Add it to the pan at the end of cooking if your food starts to burn. With a spatula or spoon, scrape up the little bits of meat or vegetable that are stuck to the pan.

Chicken and Snow Pea Stir-fry

Here's a great example both of simplicity in a recipe and of tastiness without soy sauce. In fact, the sage gives this dish a flavor reminiscent of Thanksgiving. Feel free to reduce the meat and bulk up the vegetables for a lighter meal.

2	tablespoons canola oil, divided
2	cups trimmed and cut snow peas (about 6 ounces)
6	white mushrooms, sliced
4	scallions, chopped
1/2	teaspoon salt, divided
3/4	teaspoon rubbed sage, divided
1	pound boneless, skinless chicken breast, cut into thin, bite-sized pieces

1. Heat a large skillet over high heat. Add 1 tablespoon canola oil and heat. Add snow peas, stirring quickly to coat with oil. Continue cooking about 2 minutes. Add mushrooms and scallions. Sprinkle vegetables with about half the salt and sage. Stir and cook about 1 more minute. Reduce heat to medium-high and remove vegetables. Keep warm.

2. Add remaining 1 tablespoon canola oil and allow it to heat. Add chicken. Sprinkle with remaining salt and sage. Stir and continue to cook 3–4 minutes or until chicken is cooked through, which depends on the size of your chicken pieces.

3. Return vegetables to the pan. Stir to mix well. Serve with brown rice, farro, quinoa, or any favorite grain.

Yield: about 4 1/2 cups. Serves: 4. Serving Size: 1 heaping cup.
Exchanges/Choices: 1/2 Vegetable, 3 Lean Meat, 1 1/2 Fat
Calories: 225
Total Fat: 10g/ Saturated Fat: 1g/ Trans Fat: 0g/ Cholesterol: 73mg/ Sodium: 432mg/
Total Carbohydrate: 6g/ Dietary Fiber: 2g/ Sugars: 3g/ Protein: 26g

Stir-fry Beef with Carrots and Spinach

Use jarred ginger, packaged shredded carrots, and presliced, lean stir-fry beef to save even more time.

2   **tablespoons reduced-sodium soy sauce**

1   **tablespoon sugar**

2   **teaspoons jarred or freshly grated ginger**

5   **teaspoons canola oil, divided (1 tablespoon + 2 teaspoons)**

2   **cups shredded carrots**

12   **ounces thinly sliced lean top round steak**

9-ounce bag baby spinach

Yield: about 5 cups. Serves: 4.
Serving Size: 1 heaping cup.
Exchanges/Choices: 1 Vegetable, 3 Lean Meat, 1 Fat
Calories: 233
Total Fat: 10g/ Saturated Fat: 2g/
Trans Fat: 0g/ Cholesterol: 56mg/
Sodium: 402mg/
Total Carbohydrate: 11g/ Dietary
Fiber: 3g/ Sugars: 6g/ Protein: 23g

1. Mix reduced-sodium soy sauce, sugar, and ginger together in a small bowl and set aside.

2. Heat a large skillet over high heat. Add 2 teaspoons canola oil and heat. Add shredded carrots, stirring quickly to coat with oil. Continue cooking about 1–2 minutes. Reduce heat to medium-high and remove carrots. Keep warm.

3. Add remaining 1 tablespoon canola oil and allow it to heat. Add beef. Using tongs or a spatula, stir while cooking about 2 minutes or until meat is cooked through. Be careful not to overcook meat.

4. Give soy sauce mixture a quick stir and add to the pan. Stir. Turn heat to low. Return carrots to pan and stir. Add spinach, stirring continuously to wilt. Spinach should reduce in volume by half or more.

5. Serve with tongs or slotted spoon to drain excess liquid that cooked off from spinach. Serve with brown rice, farro, quinoa, or any favorite grain.

Recipes on the Ready

Here are several ideas for throw-together meals, perfect for those nights when you come home too late to prepare the meal you had planned. Put these on your meal-planning calendar too for those days that you know you'll be crunched for time. The keys to making good use of these ideas are: 1) having staple items in your pantry, refrigerator, and freezer; and 2) remembering to go to them rather than ordering takeout or hitting the drive-thru. Make these recipes your own by using your favorite ingredients and by serving the portions appropriate for your weight, blood glucose control, etc.

Salmon Salad

Drain a can of salmon and toss with thawed broccoli florets from your freezer. Add drained and chopped marinated artichoke hearts. Add any of the following if you have them: diced red onion, diced bell pepper, and drained and rinsed canned chickpeas. Dress with olive oil and rice vinegar or your favorite Italian salad dressing. Serve with crackers or pita bread and a piece of fruit.

Salmon and Rice Salad

Drain a can of salmon and toss with leftover brown rice, quinoa, farro, or other favorite whole grain. Add chopped carrots, bell pepper, onion, or whatever is in your refrigerator. Dress with ready-made or homemade vinaigrette. Serve with sliced fresh tomato and a piece of fruit.

Pasta with Clam Sauce

Heat a jar of pasta sauce with a drained can of clams. Serve over whole-grain spaghetti and sprinkle with Parmesan cheese. Round out your meal with a bagged salad.

Tuna Melt

Drain a can of tuna and mix with just enough light mayonnaise to moisten the tuna. Add black pepper and anything else you typically like in tuna salad (pickle relish, chopped celery, or onion, for example). Place a slice of tomato on a toasted English muffin. Top it with a mound of the tuna and a slice of reduced-fat Swiss cheese. Place the muffin in the oven or toaster oven until warmed through. Broil about 1 minute to melt the cheese. Serve with a piece of fruit, bagged salad, or both.

Mediterranean Tuna Salad

Chop marinated artichoke hearts, jarred roasted bell peppers, and Kalamata olives. Mix with drained canned tuna. Season with black pepper and capers. Dress with lemon juice and olive oil. Serve with whole-grain crackers or pita bread and a piece of fruit.

Egg Burrito

Place scrambled eggs, salsa, and a sprinkling of reduced-fat Cheddar cheese into a whole-grain tortilla. Wrap and warm for a few seconds in the microwave. Serve with a fresh or frozen green vegetable and a piece of fruit.

Eggless Salad

Thoroughly drain and mash extra-firm tofu. Add chopped carrots and scallions. Mix with light mayonnaise and seasonings such as mustard, dill, onion and garlic powders, salt, and pepper. If you have some, add turmeric for the egg-yolk color. Serve with whole-grain crackers or pita bread and a piece of fruit.

Two-Bean Burrito

Mix the following into a bowl and pour into a casserole dish that's been sprayed with nonstick cooking spray: 1 can each: vegetarian refried beans; diced tomatoes, drained (preferably an unsalted variety); kidney beans, drained and rinsed; sliced black olives; and 1–2 ounces reduced-fat Cheddar cheese. Bake until heated through. Serve with whole-grain tortillas, nonfat Greek yogurt or sour cream, and jarred salsa.

Burrito Bowl

Have family members individualize their own bowls. Make each of the following (or similar) items available: prepared brown rice, drained and rinsed canned beans, diced tomatoes, diced onions, diced peppers, sliced black olives, sliced jalapeños, diced avocado, reduced-fat shredded cheese, jarred salsa, and leftover or prepared chicken or beef.

Vegetable Bean Soup

Sauté diced onions and bell peppers (either fresh or frozen). Dice and sauté any fresh vegetable you have on hand. Add drained and rinsed canned beans, undrained no-salt-added canned tomatoes, reduced-sodium chicken or vegetable broth, and Italian seasonings. Bring to a boil. Cover and simmer. Serve with whole-grain crackers or rolls and a piece of fruit.

Rotisserie Chicken

Pick up a rotisserie chicken at the supermarket. Serve with small microwaved baking potatoes, a frozen vegetable, and a bagged salad.

Salsa Chicken

Shred meat from a rotisserie chicken and place it into a saucepan with jarred salsa. Heat thoroughly. Serve over rice or with whole-grain tortillas.

Scooped French Bread Pizza

Slice a loaf of French bread lengthwise and scoop out the doughy center. Cut each half into 6–8 slices and place on a cookie sheet. Fill each cavity with sliced fresh tomatoes or a spoonful of jarred sauce. Then pick your cheese and toppings. Try baby spinach, arugula, mushrooms, or any favorite veggie. Top with reduced-fat mozzarella cheese or sprinkle with feta or goat cheese. Bake at 400°F until heated through and cheese is melted. Serve with canned soup such as lentil or tomato.

Lettuce Wraps

Whatever you would throw between two slices of bread, throw onto a big lettuce leaf and wrap. Think tuna, salmon, turkey, and chicken. Serve with fruit.

Cottage Cheese Parfait

For a sweet parfait, layer reduced-fat cottage cheese with berries and other diced fruit. Sprinkle with cinnamon. Serve with toast and peanut butter. For a savory parfait, layer reduced-fat cottage cheese with diced cucumbers, bell peppers, tomatoes, red onion, and fresh or dried herbs. Serve with whole-grain crackers.

Veggies, Beans, and Grains

There are an infinite number of ways to create a delicious meal with any favorite vegetables, beans, and grains. Simply sauté or roast any vegetables you have on hand. Mix them with a can of drained and rinsed beans (such as chickpeas or black beans) and serve over wheat berries, whole-grain couscous, quinoa, or a grain of your choice.

❧ Roasting Vegetables

If you haven't roasted vegetables, you are in for a surprise. The roasting brings out the sweetness of the vegetable, and the preparation is super fast. Follow these four steps.

1. Cut one type or a variety of vegetables into equal-size pieces. If you have vegetables that require different cooking times, however, cut the slower-cooking vegetable (such as carrots) into smaller pieces than the faster-cooking vegetable (such as zucchini).

2. Toss the vegetables with a little oil and seasonings of your choice.

3. Spread them onto a roasting pan. Don't crowd the pan or they will steam instead of roast. If necessary, use more than one pan.

4. Bake at 425°F until done. For example, green beans may take about 12 minutes, but Brussels sprouts or beets may require about 25 minutes.

Dressed-Up Grilled Cheese Sandwich

Be creative with breads, cheeses, and other fillings. Heat in a Panini press or on the stove. Try these combinations:

❧ reduced-fat Cheddar cheese with apple slices

❧ reduced-fat Havarti or Swiss cheese with strawberry slices

❧ reduced-fat mozzarella cheese with fresh tomatoes and basil

❧ turkey with reduced-fat Swiss cheese, baby spinach, and a drizzle of Italian salad dressing

- reduced-fat American cheese with sliced tomato, sliced red onion, and baby spinach

- goat cheese with sliced apples and baby spinach

Serve with reduced-sodium canned soup or a bagged salad.

Main Dish Salads

It's time to think of salads as something more than lettuce and a few vegetables. Start with salad greens, but fill in with whatever you have on hand:

- chopped onions, carrots, peppers, cucumbers, tomatoes, and other veggies

- marinated artichoke hearts, olives, corn, and marinated mushrooms

- drained and rinsed canned beans, tuna, or salmon

- hard-boiled eggs, sliced turkey or chicken, leftover steak, reduced-fat cheese

- sliced strawberries, diced apples, mandarin oranges, dried cherries

Serve with whole-grain crackers or bread.

Cookbooks for the Busy

There are many cookbooks written with speed in mind. Here are a few of my favorites:

- *Cooking Light Complete Meals in Minutes*

- *Diabetic Meals in 30 Minutes—Or Less!* by Robyn Webb

- *Quick and Healthy* by Brenda Ponichtera

- *15-Minute Diabetic Meals* by Nancy Hughes

- *Weeknight Wonders* by Ellie Krieger

Part 2:

50 EASY-TO-IMPLEMENT STRATEGIES FOR BETTER HEALTH

The *Overworked Person's Guide to Better Nutrition* is written for people with hectic lives, but it is not only about timesaving strategies. Though you will learn to do more in less time, some tips are simply bare-bones explanations of important health topics. They are mini nutrition and health lessons. I am including the same information I teach to my patients, but it is streamlined so that every day or every week, you have just the right information and the right amount of it to get started on a new, healthy behavior. As I've said earlier, it's smart to focus on the tips and strategies that are most meaningful to you. You'll save time and make more headway.

First of all, it's important to consider both willpower and habits. Most people think that they don't have enough willpower but that others are blessed with ample amounts of it. Or they think that they've had willpower in the past but have regained lost weight, or watched their blood glucose or cholesterol rise, because their willpower failed them. The myth of willpower is the undoing of many dieters and others trying to improve their health. Trust me—nobody has enough willpower to eat or behave exactly as they wish they did all of the time, from now until forever. No one. Those who are successful at long-term weight control, blood glucose management, or other significant diet or lifestyle changes use strategies and develop skills. Willpower fades when we get bored with our diet plan, or feel deprived, or when we have extra stress in our lives. If you've lost weight or improved your cholesterol or glucose levels because you strictly followed a rigid diet plan only to later undo all that you achieved, you were probably relying on willpower to get to your goal. Unlike willpower, skills and strategies can last forever. It's not about trying harder; it's about trying smarter.

Eventually, these skills and strategies lead you to good habits. Habits make our lives easier. The brain doesn't have to work as hard once you know how to tie your shoe or drive to work, or know to brush your teeth when getting ready for bed. The steps to doing these things are habitual; they are ingrained in your mind, so you do not need as much mental energy to get them done. Conserving mental energy through habits is especially important the more overworked and busy you are. The notion that it takes 21 days to form a habit is another myth. The length of time it takes depends on many factors, including the desired behavior, the degree of difficulty, and multiple individual and environmental factors. According to the results of one study, it took from

18 to 254 days to form a new health-related habit. To work toward new habits such as strength training, measuring your blood glucose after meals, or flossing your teeth, pick a very manageable goal, attach it to an existing behavior, then do it daily—not now and then, but at least once daily. For example, when I had trouble remembering to floss my teeth, I decided to link it to my shower, since a shower is a daily activity. Every time I showered, I flossed. I didn't even force myself to floss all of my teeth (though I usually did), but I forced myself to do something. Eventually, flossing became such a habit that if I took two showers in one day, I had to force myself not to floss the second time. Use this technique for any desired habit, but be sure to emphasize small. In fact, it's better to err on the small side than to pick something unmanageable. If your ultimate goal is to exercise daily for 30 minutes, it's okay to start with just 5 minutes. If full-body strength training is your goal, start with 1 minute of sit-ups and 1 minute of push-ups, for example.

Once you have your habit, guard it carefully. It's easy to fall out of a routine, and not always simple to regain it. Even when your routine must change, try to maintain as much of it as possible. If you are injured and cannot run, for instance, spend at least a few minutes walking, biking, or stretching. Or if your work schedule temporarily changes, leaving you without 30 minutes to walk at lunchtime, walk for 5 minutes instead. You'll be in the same walking habit once your usual schedule resumes.

I recently learned about Tiny Habits®. Run by its creator, BJ Fogg, PhD, director of the Persuasive Tech Lab at Stanford University, this program helps people form new habits by having them perform the desired behavior or a piece of the desired behavior for no more than 30 seconds. For example, if you want to acquire the habit of meditating after breakfast, you can start by simply sitting in a meditative position for 30 seconds every day after breakfast. You can learn more about Tiny Habits® or sign up for a free 5-day session at tinyhabits.com.

Chapter 3:

EAT MORE

Nature provides an abundance of healthful foods that together feed us lifesaving nutrients. This chapter takes the *what-to-eat* approach and teaches you to incorporate nature's best into your daily diet. Eating ample power foods does double duty: it ensures that you're getting an arsenal of disease-fighting nutrients, and it makes less room in the belly for the less desirable foods. Don't worry though—even the best diets can accommodate your favorites, no matter what they are!

Health-Boosting Strategy #1

Love the limas. Grab the great northerns.

Beans, beans—they really are good for your heart, and a lot else. So what if they have that gas thing going on? There's so much in their favor that beans should be at the top of your shopping list. They're inexpensive, versatile, and pack a nutritional punch. Beans and other legumes offer as much as 16 grams of fiber and 20 grams of protein per cup, with healthy doses of folate, potassium, magnesium, and resistant starch as well. (See Health-Boosting Strategy #4 for more on resistant starches.)

According to a study of nearly 10,000 men and women, eating at least four servings of beans per week—compared to eating beans less than once weekly—lowers the risk of coronary heart disease by 22%. Can beans give you more birthdays? Maybe. Researchers studying longevity in four countries found that the consumption of legumes was the greatest dietary predictor of survival among the elderly.

What other health benefits can beans claim?

⚬ Beans may slow tumor growth and prevent tumor cells from reproducing.

⚬ Bean eaters tend to have trimmer waistlines and are less likely to be obese than non-bean eaters. Beans' high fiber content may tame hunger.

⚬ Compounds in beans may help improve blood cholesterol, blood pressure, and blood glucose.

According to the U.S. Department of Health and Human Services/U.S. Department of Agriculture (USDA) *Dietary Guidelines for Americans*, most of us should eat at least 1 1/2 cups of legumes each week. Baked beans, bean salads, and chili are a few favorite legume-rich dishes, but they probably won't get you to 1 1/2 cups a week, every week. Time to get creative.

⚬ Snack on hummus and whole-grain crackers.

⚬ Spread hummus instead of mayonnaise on a sandwich.

⚬ Make a meatless three-bean chili with pintos, black beans, and kidney beans.

⚬ Extend your ground meat with lentils.

⚬ Start a meal or have a snack with edamame beans. Boil frozen edamame beans still in their pods. Sprinkle lightly with coarse salt, if desired.

⚬ Add black beans to a tomato-basil sauce and serve over whole-wheat pasta.

⚬ For a quick salad or topping for grilled fish or chicken, rinse canned black beans and corn. Toss them with your favorite jarred salsa. Add fresh cilantro if you have it.

⚬ Toss rinsed, canned beans into your mixed green salad. Each week, try a different type of bean.

- Fancy up tuna salad with garbanzos and fresh herbs.

- Add canned beans to prepared soups.

- Thicken chili, stews, and soups with puréed or smashed white beans. (Smash them well, and I promise that no one will know they are there.)

- Mix red beans into store-bought or homemade pasta salad.

- Top tortilla chips with kidney beans and reduced-fat cheese. Microwave briefly. Then add a dollop of nonfat Greek yogurt and jarred salsa.

Don't fear beans because of their well-deserved reputation for causing gas. Instead, move gradually to a high-fiber diet to allow your body time to adjust. Discarding the liquid from canned or presoaked beans rids your plate of some of the hard-to-digest, noxious carbohydrates. Finally, consider an over-the-counter aid like Beano to help digest the offending carbohydrates.

Get It Fast Tips

Split peas and lentils, especially red lentils, cook up super fast. And using a pressure cooker will give you other cooked beans in a fraction of the time that traditional cooking takes.

BONUS TIPS

- Drain and rinse canned beans to wash away about 40% of the sodium.

- When cooking with dried beans, sort through them carefully. Spread them out on a towel of contrasting color to identify and remove dirt and debris. Then rinse the remaining beans before soaking. Quick soak method: Cover the beans with cold water. Boil for 2–3 minutes. Remove the pot from the heat and leave it covered for 1 hour. Drain and rinse with fresh cold water. Now the beans are ready to cook.

Health-Boosting Strategy #2

Punch up the flavor with phytochemical-packed herbs and spices.

Sprinkling herbs and spices on food reduces the need for salt. But there is more: these flavor-packed seasonings can raise everyday cooking from good to great and give you an additional health boost along the way. Like fruits and vegetables, herbs and spices are loaded with phytochemicals. These plant compounds provide color and aroma while protecting the plant from attacks by insects and disease. In the diet, phytochemicals work together with other nutrients to protect us from disease. Though research on the topic is still ongoing, compounds in herbs and spices may help shield our health in any of the following ways. They may:

- act as an antioxidant or antimicrobial

- reduce pain

- fight cancer

- improve blood vessel function

- reduce blood cholesterol

- control blood glucose

Though it's all a matter of taste, use the following chart to get started.

SEASONING	USES & NOTES
Basil	Fresh tomatoes, tomato dishes, soups and stews, salads, rice, poultry, fish, beef, Italian cuisine *Fresh basil is much tastier than dried basil. It's very delicate, so add it after cooking. Slip a few leaves inside a sandwich.*
Cardamom	Breads, fruit, chicken, rice, spiced coffee; Middle Eastern and Indian cuisines *Cardamom pairs nicely with cinnamon. Add it early in the cooking process.*
Chile pepper	Beans, bell peppers, corn, rice, potatoes, beef, chicken, chocolate; Mexican and Thai cuisines *Add chile peppers at the end of the cooking process.*
Cilantro	Tomatoes, green salads, avocados, black beans, lentils, chutneys, salsas, rice; Mexican, Thai, and Indian cuisines *Cilantro pairs well with chile peppers. Fresh cilantro is tastier than dried. Its flavor and leaves are delicate, so add them after cooking.*
Cinnamon	Breads, fruit, winter squash, chicken, lamb, chocolate, nuts, coffee, tea; Moroccan and Indian cuisines *Add cinnamon early in the cooking process.*
Dill	Cucumbers, beets, carrots, tomatoes, eggs, salads, green vegetables, potatoes, fish and fish sauces, yogurt and yogurt sauces *Add dill after cooking.*
Mint	Cucumbers, carrots, eggplant, tomatoes, salads, sauces and dips, peas, lamb, melon and other fruit, yogurt; Middle Eastern and Mediterranean cuisines *Fresh mint is tastier than dried. Add mint after cooking.*
Oregano	Bell peppers, tomatoes, eggplant, mushrooms, olives, onions, zucchini, salads, soups and stews, beef, lamb; Italian and Greek cuisines *Add oregano toward the end of cooking.*

SEASONING	USES & NOTES
Rosemary	Bell peppers, eggplant, mushrooms, tomatoes, green vegetables, potatoes, soups and stews, beef, poultry, pork, shrimp; French and Italian cuisines *Rosemary has a robust flavor, so add fresh or dried rosemary early in the cooking process.*
Thyme	Tomatoes, green beans, carrots, eggplant, parsnips, zucchini, salads, beef, poultry, eggs, fish, lamb *Add dried or fresh thyme early in the cooking process.*

Primer on Herbs and Spices

Store dried seasonings in a cabinet or drawer away from light, heat, and moisture. Pour them into your hand or a spoon instead of shaking the bottle over a hot pot, because the steam from the pot can enter the bottle and cause the seasonings' flavor to deteriorate. Dried herbs usually have a more concentrated flavor, so substitute one part dried herbs for three parts fresh (for example, 1 teaspoon dried for 1 tablespoon fresh). Keep fresh-cut herbs in the refrigerator. Place their stems in a jar of water, and cover the leaves with a plastic bag. Change the water approximately every other day. I so love fresh herbs in cooking and salads that I want to have them on hand always. In the warm months, I grow them outside, but once the weather turns cold, I use my AeroGarden (aerogrow.com) indoors.

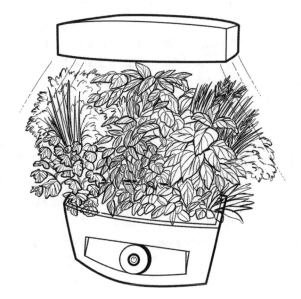

Don't forget premixed spice blends to save both time and money. Read labels on these, as on any other food. You might be very surprised by just how much sodium is in blends such as lemon pepper and Italian seasonings. If you're new to cooking without salt or if you're trying out new herbs and spices, consider these premixed blends in their salt-free varieties:

- lemon pepper

- Italian medley

- garlic and herb

- chipotle, Cajun, or jerk

- Caribbean

Health-Boosting Strategy #3

Sneak fruits and vegetables into the foods you already eat—every day.

You probably already know that good health requires eating ample fruits and vegetables. As a nation, we consume only 59% of the recommended amount of vegetables. We do even worse with fruit, meeting only 42% of the target intake, according to the *Dietary Guidelines for Americans*. Instead of revamping your entire diet (unless it truly needs revamping), increase your intake of fruits and vegetables by adding them to the foods you currently eat. It's simple to toss chopped celery and sliced grapes into your usual chicken salad, or diced carrots and zucchini into spaghetti sauce. There are plenty of suggestions below to add fruits and vegetables to recipes or to prepare them in new ways.

So why eat more? Fruits and vegetables provide several underconsumed nutrients, including dietary fiber, potassium, magnesium, folate, and vitamins A, C, and K. In addition, they are loaded with phytochemicals, natural plant compounds that act synergistically in the body with thousands of other phytochemicals and nutrients to shield us from disease. Because each fruit and vegetable provides a unique array of phytochemicals, limiting yourself to just a few favorite fruits and vegetables limits your diet's health-shielding powers.

A diet rich in fruits and vegetables is linked to lower blood pressure, less stroke, less coronary heart disease, and reduced risks of type 2 diabetes, obesity, and certain cancers. According to the joint expert report from the American Institute for Cancer Research and the World Cancer Research Fund, diets rich in fruits and vegetables are linked to lower risks of cancers of the mouth, pharynx, larynx, esophagus, lung, pancreas, prostate, and stomach. The federal government's MyPlate advises women to consume at least 1 1/2 cups of fruit and 2 cups of vegetables daily. Men should eat at least 2 cups of fruit and 2 1/2 cups of vegetables each day. To learn more, visit ChooseMyPlate.gov.

If you need to get closer to targets, pick a few of the following strategies to help. Plan to eat a fruit and/or vegetable with every meal and snack.

- Fill an omelet with vegetables like chopped tomatoes, onions, mushrooms, and peppers. Or top scrambled eggs with a favorite jarred salsa.

- Add shredded carrots or zucchini to ground meat before shaping into a meatloaf or meatballs.

- Stuff sandwiches with more veggies than meat. Go for bell peppers, mushrooms, avocado, red onion, and spinach.

- Brighten up a green salad with fresh and dried fruits.

- Add diced cauliflower, broccoli, or tomatoes to casseroles like lasagna and macaroni and cheese.

- Purée cooked cauliflower and mix with mashed potatoes.

- Add zucchini, green beans, or eggplant to any favorite jarred spaghetti sauce.

- Stir puréed pumpkin or winter squash into chili or tomato-based casseroles.

- Add canned or frozen vegetables to soups.

✌ Eat double servings of vegetables at dinner.

✌ Top a baked potato with beans and salsa. Better yet, offer your family a potato bar. Everyone gets a baked potato and a choice of several toppings such as scallions, steamed broccoli, sautéed bell peppers, chopped tomato, jarred salsa, drained and rinsed canned beans, diced avocado, sautéed mushrooms, diced chicken, reduced-fat shredded cheese, reduced-fat cottage cheese, and nonfat Greek yogurt.

✌ Dip raw veggies into hummus or salsa.

✌ Toss nonfat yogurt and your favorite frozen fruits into a blender for a quick smoothie. For a green smoothie, add a celery stick and a handful of baby spinach.

✌ Thread pineapple, peaches, peppers, mushrooms, and cherry tomatoes on skewers to toss on the grill.

✌ Mix diced tomatoes and herbs from the garden with reduced-fat cottage cheese, or try raisins and cinnamon or blueberries and almonds.

✌ Skewer up fresh berries, grapes, and peach slices for a fun dessert.

✌ Slice nectarines, bananas, strawberries, or other fresh fruit onto cereal.

✌ Enjoy frozen fruits straight from the freezer for a cooling treat.

✌ Grill fruit for dessert or for a sweet side dish.

🌿 Get It Fast Tips

Buy fresh produce in small quantities, so it doesn't spoil before you've had a chance to eat it. Even though bananas come in bunches, you can buy just one, and you can pull out just a few handfuls of grapes or cherries from a large open bag at the market. If time is precious (and I know that it is), seek out convenience. Buy a variety of canned and frozen fruits and vegetables to limit your trips to the supermarket. Look for individual servings of frozen vegetables that you can microwave for lunch. Most supermarkets offer bagged salads, ready-to-microwave fresh vegetables, and a variety of precut fruits and vegetables. Some even have salad bars from which you can take small amounts of broccoli, cauliflower, mushrooms, and other precut produce to use in recipes. Once at home, portion out individual servings of grapes, cherries, or raw veggies into small plastic bags to make it as easy to grab a wholesome snack as it is to grab a bag of chips.

BONUS TIPS

🌿 Take fruit to work to beat the afternoon slump. You'll boost your health and beat the 3:00 slowdown at the same time. Each Monday, before leaving the house for work, grab five fruits, one for each afternoon. Get the most nutrition by going for variety. Consider the color palette—green (kiwi), red (cherries), white/brown (banana), yellow/orange (apricot), blue/purple (plum)—and type, such as stone fruits (peach), berries (strawberries), melon (cantaloupe), citrus (clementine), and others.

🌿 If fruit alone isn't enough to prevent the slump, add reduced-fat cheese or cottage cheese, nuts, deli-sliced turkey, or some food that is missing from your meals.

🌿 If you fall into a slump most afternoons, your lunch or breakfast may be the culprit. See Health-Boosting Strategy #27 for more information. And don't forget the exercise. Yes, it boosts energy. Even if all you have is 2 or 3 minutes, take them. Walk quickly, stretch, do a few jumping jacks; anything is better than nothing, and it all helps!

Health-Boosting Strategy #4

Don't resist resistant starches.

As their name suggests, these carbohydrates resist digestion in the small intestine. Since they are neither digested nor absorbed, they do not contribute to blood glucose levels—a plus for people with diabetes and prediabetes. But their real benefit comes when resistant starches reach the colon, where they serve as food for our gut bacteria. Intestinal bacteria—and we carry about 3 pounds of them—make a meal out of the resistant starch; in the process, they produce fatty acids that make the environment more suitable for the good bacteria and less suitable for the bad guys. These good bacteria have many roles. They produce vitamins, detoxify cancer-causing compounds, and activate health-promoting compounds. The fatty acids also promote healthy colon cells and may even improve the body's response to insulin. Resistant starches may help you control your weight too. Some studies suggest that they increase satiety— the feeling of fullness. So how can you get more resistant starches in your diet? Try to eat the following foods and similar choices, such as other beans, often.

FOOD	RESISTANT STARCH (GRAMS)
White beans, 1 cup cooked	7.4
Lentils, 1 cup cooked	6.8
Underripe banana, 1 medium	4.7
Rolled oats, 1/4 cup, uncooked	4.4
Potato, cooked then cooled, 3 1/2 ounces	4.3
Chickpeas, 1 cup cooked	4.0
Kidney beans, 1 cup cooked	2.8
Green peas, 1/2 cup cooked	2.0
Pearl barley, 1/2 cup cooked	1.9
Puffed wheat cereal, 1 ounce	1.7
Brown rice, 1/2 cup cooked	1.6
Quinoa, 1/2 cup cooked	1.0
Pumpernickel bread, 1 ounce	1.3
Rye bread, 1 ounce	0.9

Cooked and chilled potatoes have more resistant starch than cooked potatoes that have not been cooled. The same is true for other starches such as rice and pasta. Enjoy potato salad and other cold starchy salads in reasonable portions. Uncooked oats are also a good source of resistant starch, but cooked oats are not, though both offer great nutrition. In just a few minutes, you can make your own muesli, a combination of uncooked oats, dried fruit, and nuts. Add wheat germ, rye flakes, brown sugar (just a little bit), cinnamon, and other flavors according to your preference. Mine is a simple combination of oats, cinnamon, raisins, and nuts. Eat muesli with cottage cheese, Greek yogurt, or with a splash of nonfat or low-fat milk for a super-fast, nutrient-packed breakfast.

In addition to choosing foods rich in naturally occurring resistant starches, you can add Hi-maize® resistant starch to baked goods, yogurt, cottage cheese, and smoothies or seek out pasta, breads, and other packaged foods with added resistant starches. For more information, visit the Hi-maize® website at http://www.hi-maize.com.

Health-Boosting Strategy #5

Drink brewed, not bottled, tea for a healthy heart.

In many research studies, an association has been found between tea drinking and a reduced risk of heart attack, lowering of high blood pressure, and improved cholesterol levels. Like other edible plants, tea provides phytochemical disease fighters, especially flavonoids. According to Jeffrey Blumberg, PhD, professor of nutrition science and policy at Tufts University, drinking a cup of tea is like adding a serving of fruits or vegetables to your diet.

Unfortunately, most ready-to-drink teas, though convenient, contain little if any flavonoids. Here's how to get the most health boosters from tea:

✌ Brew tea in hot water. Tea brewed in cold or room-temperature water has less flavonoids.

✌ Brew iced tea double strength because the ice dilutes the tea and health-boosting flavonoids.

✌ Store iced tea in the refrigerator for just a day or two. The longer you store it, the more the flavonoids degrade. Have you noticed that the bottom of the pitcher gets cloudy? That's from degraded flavonoids.

✌ Add a few fresh lemon or orange slices to your iced tea pitcher. The vitamin C in citrus fruits helps protect the flavonoids from degradation.

Additional research suggests there may be even more benefits to drinking tea, such as:

✌ cancer protection

✌ brain health

- increased bone formation and muscle strength

- reduced level of stress hormones and raised mental alertness

BONUS TIP
All nonherbal teas come from the leaves of the Camellia sinensis plant. The differences between black, green, white, and oolong teas are due to how the leaves are processed. Brew black tea with boiling water, but the others are best brewed with water that is below the boiling point.

Health-Boosting Strategy #6

Go fish—at least twice weekly.

Fatty fish is good for the heart. The American Heart Association and the American Diabetes Association recommend eating fish at least twice weekly, preferably salmon and other fish—including trout, mackerel, bluefish, herring, sardines, halibut, and tuna—that are rich in the omega-3 fatty acids DHA and EPA. Research suggests that these fatty acids decrease the risk of abnormal heartbeats, slow the progression of plaque in the arteries, and improve blood triglycerides. Other research has found that these omega-3 fatty acids help to prevent or slow the progression of cognitive decline during aging, dementia, and age-related eye disease and help slow or prevent other health conditions.

You can buy fresh and frozen fish at your supermarket or fish market. Though it may be the easiest and quickest choice to get, skip breaded and fried fish. This cooking method is less healthy, and the types of fish that are typically breaded and fried are not rich in omega-3 fatty acids.

- Place a salmon fillet in the oven. When it's done, dress it with a mixture of olive oil, lemon juice, garlic, and fresh basil (a favorite in my house) or any flavorful vinaigrette.

- Brush a fish fillet with olive oil and sprinkle with chopped fresh herbs before baking or grilling.

Get It Fast Tips

For the sake of convenience, keep individually wrapped frozen fillets and easy-to-peel shrimp on hand. Thaw them quickly in a sealed plastic bag placed into a pot or bowl of cold water. Fortunately, shrimp and most fish are quick and easy to prepare.

- Open a can for a quick tuna or salmon salad. See Chapter 2 on pages 37 and 38 for some ideas.

- Add sardines to a salad or eat them with whole-grain crackers.

- Spread jarred pesto sauce over a fish fillet before cooking.

- After brushing fish with olive oil or light mayonnaise, press chopped nuts or seasoned bread crumbs onto your fillet. Then bake.

- Quickly and simply cook salmon and shrimp in parchment paper. See Chapter 2 on pages 31 and 32 for recipes.

Most fish should be cooked to an internal temperature of 145°F. It's helpful to have an instant-read thermometer for measuring doneness. Additionally, fish fillets should be opaque and flaky. Shrimp and lobster should look opaque and pearly. And scallops become opaque and firm when thoroughly cooked.

Purchasing Seafood

- Buy fresh fish or shellfish only if it's refrigerated or on a thick bed of ice that is not melting.

- Frozen seafood should be in a sealed package. It should not show frost or ice crystals.

🐟 Fresh fish should smell fresh and mild. The flesh should be firm, moist, and shiny with even coloring. When you press the flesh with your finger, it should spring back.

🐟 Shrimp flesh should be shiny and translucent.

Seafood Safety

Are you concerned about the mercury and PCBs (polychlorinated biphenyls) in fish? Though both are undesirable contaminants in fish, they should not deter you from enjoying seafood in reasonable amounts. Mercury occurs naturally in the environment and is also released into the air through industrial pollution. Fish absorb the mercury, which accumulates in the oceans and streams. PCBs are toxic industrial compounds that have been banned from use for more than three decades. However, they are slow to break down, and they build up in the fish that live in contaminated water. The Environmental Protection Agency (EPA) and the U.S. Food and Drug Administration (FDA) recommend the following:

🐟 Women who are pregnant, may become pregnant, or are breast-feeding, and children up to age 12, should not eat the following four fish because of their high mercury content: shark, swordfish, tilefish, and king mackerel. This group of women can safely consume 12 ounces of other fish per week with no more than 6 ounces of white (albacore) tuna per week. Canned light tuna has less mercury than white (albacore) tuna. Children can eat the same fish, but their portions should be smaller.

🐟 Healthy adolescents and most adults will benefit from choosing a variety of seafood. If eating fish more than twice weekly, eat a variety of types to reduce the risk of contaminants from a single source.

Sustainable Seafood

To learn about sustainable choices, visit the website of the Monterey Bay Aquarium (montereybayaquarium.org). There you can read about ocean-friendly seafood, download a consumer pocket guide, or get an app for iPhone or Android phones.

Health-Boosting Strategy #7

Keep nutritious foods in view.

If you want to eat more of something, put it where you'll see it. That's the advice of my patient, Sharon, who has lost considerable weight and improved her diabetes control and cholesterol levels. It seems so simple, yet many people don't think of doing it. Sharon keeps raw vegetables and vegetable juice in an obvious place in the refrigerator with the idea that she'll see these first and reach for them instead of something less nutritious.

I used this logic when my children were young. Just before they came home from school, I'd put a bowl of fresh fruit on the kitchen table where they dumped their backpacks and started their homework. They usually ate the fruit with little verbal prompting. It was a subtle way of helping them make a wise choice, and it kept arguments about food to a minimum.

Health-Boosting Strategy #8

Go vegetarian now and then.

A plant-based diet—simply described, one that contains more foods of plant origin than of animal origin—nourishes your body with vitamins, minerals, fiber, and thousands of phytochemicals that are protective of heart disease, type 2 diabetes, metabolic syndrome, some cancers, and other chronic health problems. There are many versions of a healthful plant-based diet. Some may include fish or eggs, dairy, and even pork and beef, or others may include none of these. A diet with no animal products at all is called a vegan diet. I like the plant-based diet described by the American Institute for Cancer Research (aicr.org) because of its simplicity and because it is doable for most people.

Called the New American Plate, it emphasizes both portion and proportion. Make the proportion of food from plant sources much greater than the proportion of food from animal sources. Plan your meals so that at least two-thirds of your intake comes from vegetables, fruits, grains, beans, and nuts and no more than one-third of your food comes from meats and dairy. Doing so assures you a flood of health-boosting nutrients and phytochemicals as long as your choices are wise and not based on overly processed foods. Be smart about portion sizes too to help manage your weight, which in turn affects your risk for disease.

Many people are jumping on the Meatless Monday bandwagon because it's a valuable yet manageable commitment to limiting their meat intake. Learn more about Meatless Monday at meatlessmonday.com.

🥕 Get It Fast Tips

For a quick, meatless breakfast, mix fruit into Greek yogurt or cottage cheese. Lunch on canned lentil or black bean soup or a plate of edamame beans. For dinner, mix a can of vegetarian refried beans with salsa, chopped scallions, and drained and rinsed kidney beans. Sprinkle with reduced-fat cheese, and heat the mixture thoroughly before wrapping a few large spoonfuls with a whole-grain tortilla. More meatless meals: stir-fry tofu with frozen vegetables or toss a frozen veggie burger onto the grill or into the microwave.

HINT: To learn more about plant-based diets, take a look at *The Plant-Powered Diet*, written by my friend and colleague Sharon Palmer, RD. One of Sharon's tips is to convert your favorite recipes into meatless ones. For example, if you have a favorite lasagna, skip the meat and pile on the veggies. Or if taco night is a family favorite, omit the ground beef and substitute meatless crumbles, beans, and lots of vegetables including tomatoes, green onions, lettuce, avocado, and cilantro.

Health-Boosting Strategy #9

Join team lutein. Eat spinach, kale, and corn for healthy eyes and brain.

Snack on kale chips. Grill corn for dinner, and throw a handful of raw spinach into your morning smoothie. Lutein and zeaxanthin, found in these foods and others, protect your eyes and brain. The two compounds are relatives of beta-carotene and are members of the carotenoid family of phytochemicals. What makes lutein and zeaxanthin so valuable is that they are the only carotenoids to make their way into the macula of the eye, where they are present in high concentrations. Constantly being exposed to light, the macula is subject to oxidative damage, but luckily for us, lutein and zeaxanthin are there acting as both antioxidants and a light filter. Eating foods rich in lutein and zeaxanthin is related to a decrease in age-related macular degeneration, the number one cause of blindness and severe vision loss in adults aged over 60 years. In this case, what's good for the eyes is good for the brain too. Lutein and zeaxanthin are also present there, and studies suggest that higher levels in the brain may protect against cognitive decline. So eat some lutein. Find it in these foods:

- spinach, kale, collard greens, and other leafy greens

- broccoli

- corn

- acorn squash and other winter squashes

- summer squash

- peas

- broccoli

- Brussels sprouts

- bell peppers

- pistachios

- egg yolks

Get It Fast Tips

- Keep frozen vegetables handy and microwave them for dinner.

- Grab a handful of frozen corn and peas; after they've defrosted, toss them into a green salad.

- To make kale chips, buy a bag of torn and ready-to-eat kale. Toss with olive oil and a very small amount of coarse salt. Add any additional flavors you like, such as garlic, paprika or chile pepper, and lime. Spread the leaves on a baking sheet in a single layer. Bake at 275°F for 20–30 minutes. Come back to the oven midway to turn the leaves. They will be crisp when done. Eat them right away; they stay crispy for just a couple of hours.

Health-Boosting Strategy #10

Find (and eat) fermented foods.

Eating fermented foods can provide your gut with the healthy bacteria (probiotics) it needs to crowd out the not-so-good bacteria. Fermented foods are made or preserved by yeast or bacteria. Research suggests that the benefits of probiotics include enhanced immune function, greater digestive health, and a lower prevalence of allergy. Fermentation may also increase the digestibility or absorption of certain nutrients. Lactose, for example, is broken down when milk becomes yogurt or kefir.

The fermentation process was traditionally used to preserve foods, so fermented foods have been around for eons. Cabbage became sauerkraut. Cucumbers became pickles. Milk became yogurt, kefir, or cottage cheese. Unfortunately, you can't count on all sauerkraut, pickles, or any food that was traditionally fermented to contain probiotics. Manufacturers frequently use nonfermentation techniques to prepare foods these days, and often, even if they do ferment the food, heating, filtering, or other processes likely kill the microorganisms.

Some fermented foods:

❧ yogurt

❧ kefir—fermented milk, similar to yogurt but drinkable

❧ cottage cheese

❧ pickles

❧ sauerkraut

❧ kimchi—spicy fermented cabbage

❧ miso—fermented soybeans, frequently used in soups, salad dressings, and marinades

❧ poi—fermented stem of the taro plant

HINT: Look for the words *live active cultures* or a similar description on packaging. Yogurt containers may bear a voluntary *Live and Active Cultures* seal from the National Yogurt Association. Find fermented vegetables like pickles and sauerkraut in the refrigerated section of your local supermarket or specialty store. They should be nonpasteurized to retain the live cultures. If you're not sure whether your favorite brand of cottage cheese, pickles, or any other food contains live cultures, call the manufacturer to ask. Check the product's expiration date and storage instructions. To retain active cultures, the product must be fresh and properly stored.

Health-Boosting Strategy #11

Replace some refined grains with whole grains.

Americans eat plenty of grains, but unfortunately, we don't eat the most healthful ones. On average, we consume only 15% of the recommended amount of whole grains, but we eat twice the recommended limit of refined grains. In fact, less than 5% of Americans consume enough whole grains. In addition to providing a host of nutrients, a diet rich in whole grains is associated with lower body weight and less heart disease, type 2 diabetes, and certain types of cancers.

A whole grain contains all three components of the grain seed: bran, germ, and endosperm. Some whole grains such as brown rice, wild rice, whole wheat, oatmeal, and rye are familiar to many. Barley, quinoa, and buckwheat are becoming more popular and more common. But there is a whole world of more exotic whole grains out there. They include amaranth, farro, millet, sorghum, and teff. To learn about them, visit the website of the Whole Grains Council (wholegrainscouncil.org). If this list of unusual whole grains doesn't interest you, that's okay. Stick with the others until your interest is piqued.

Get It Fast Tips

Since whole grains can take a long time to cook, make extra to have them on hand later. Cooked grains will keep for up to 3 days in the refrigerator or for up to 4 months in the freezer. If you're ready to rewarm frozen grains, thaw them first, then add a few tablespoons of water or broth and reheat in the microwave. You can also buy quick-cooking oats, barley, farro, and whole-grain rice.

Often products claim "made with whole grains," but this doesn't tell you much. Is the product made with a lot or a little? Reading the list of ingredients in a food helps. Quickly scan the label for these words or ingredients that indicate whole grains:

- whole in front of any grain such as whole wheat and whole rye

- brown rice, wild rice, black rice, red rice

- buckwheat

- millet

- oatmeal, oats, rolled oats

- popcorn

- quinoa

- wheat berries

These terms do not indicate whole grains:

- degerminated corn

- enriched wheat

- stone-ground: unless the word whole is also present, as in stone-ground whole wheat

- multigrain: unless the word whole is also present

An even quicker way to know if a product contains a significant amount of whole grains is to look for the Whole Grain Stamp from the Whole Grains Council. If the product contains at least 8 grams of whole grains (half of a whole-grain serving), it may bear the label. Not every company participates in this voluntary program, however. Consuming at least 48 grams of whole grains daily is ideal.

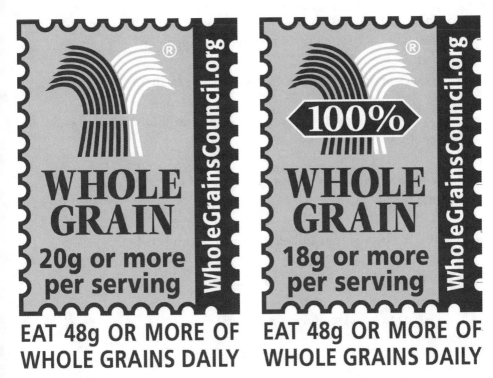

Images courtesy of Oldways and the Whole Grains Council (www.wholegrainscouncil.org).

Health-Boosting Strategy #12

Take oats beyond the bowl.

Like other whole grains, oats provide ample nutrition. Just as it's good for you to eat an array of fruits and vegetables, I hope you'll enjoy a variety of whole grains such as wheat berries, quinoa, brown rice, wild rice, buckwheat, amaranth, and farro. But oats have something most other whole grains don't have—a fiber called beta-glucan. This soluble fiber sweeps cholesterol from your digestive tract before it reaches your bloodstream. It also appears to improve insulin action and lowers blood glucose.

Enjoy oatmeal for breakfast and in many other ways:

- Thicken soups and stews with a handful of oats. Just add to the pot and cook.

- Mix oats into your ground meat when making meatballs or meatloaf. If you use steel-cut oats, soften them first in egg or egg white.

- Coat chicken or fish with seasoned oats before baking.

- Swap one-third of the flour for oats in recipes for muffins, pancakes, breads, and cookies.

- Look for recipes on the website of Quaker Oats, Bob's Red Mill, or any favorite brand.

Barley also has beta-glucan and offers similar health benefits.

- Cook up a barley pilaf in place of rice pilaf.

- Add barley to bread stuffing.

- Make your favorite pasta salad recipe with barley instead of pasta.

- Warm up with a cup of mushroom barley soup.

Get It Fast Tips

It's not just long-cooking oats that supply us with beta-glucan. Make a fast bowl of instant or quick-cooking oats for your morning dose of this health-shielding fiber. Barley too comes in a quick-cooking variety. If you prefer traditional oats and barley, consider using my method, a rice cooker. I favor it for its ease; I can walk away and do other things while my whole grains cook. When they're done, the rice cooker turns itself off. You can also eat cold oat cereal like Cheerios and find products like Sneaky Pete's Oat Beverage that have added oat fiber.

BONUS TIP
If you avoid gluten because of celiac disease or other gluten intolerance, look for gluten-free oats such as Bob's Red Mill (bobsredmill.com) and Gifts of Nature (giftsofnature.net).

Chapter 4:
EAT LESS

In this chapter, you'll learn some simple ways to trim sodium, saturated fat, added sugars, and extra calories. None of these tips will overhaul your diet, but by being consistent with these small changes, you can see meaningful results in your health, including blood pressure, blood glucose, and cholesterol levels and your weight.

Health-Boosting Strategy #13

Love the taste of water.

It's calorie-free and a perfect choice to keep you hydrated. Ditching sugary drinks in favor of water trims calories and carbs and often results in a slimmer physique. Some of my patients with diabetes have been shocked to see how much their blood glucose levels improved and even more shocked by their boost in energy, improved sleep, and disappearing headaches. If you don't already like the taste of water, dress it up with your favorite flavors. Only your creativity limits your choices. Just add fruit and herbs to a pitcher of water and refrigerate. You don't need to buy a special water pitcher or water bottle, but do so if it helps. I like these: Define Bottle (definebottle.com) and Prodyne (prodyne.com).

Try adding some of following combinations to water. A few may sound a bit odd, but they really do taste great:

- cucumber slices with mint

- cucumber slices with lavender

- lemon or oranges slices, or both

- lemon slices with grated gingerroot

- grapefruit, orange, and lime slices with mint

- peach slices with basil

- strawberry and lime slices with rosemary

- strawberry and lime slices with mint

- cubed watermelon, pineapple, and honeydew or cantaloupe

- pineapple cubes and orange slices

- blackberries and lime slices with mint

- blackberries and lime slices with basil

When adding herbs like basil and mint, gently crush them in your hand to release their flavors. Some of these flavor combinations, like the lemon- or orange-flavored water, taste delicious within a few minutes and even better in a few hours. Others such as the strawberry, rosemary, and lime need to sit refrigerated for several hours.

Get It Fast Tips

If you need a more convenient solution to flavoring your water, buy a flavor packet such as True Lemon, True Lime, or True Grapefruit. These are all natural and unsweetened packs about the size of a sugar packet. You can take them to restaurants, keep them in your wallet or gym bag, and have them handy whenever you need a flavor boost. Look for them in the supermarket baking aisle. If you want something sweet and don't object to artificial flavors and sweeteners, you have lots of choices, including Crystal Light and less expensive store brands.

Health-Boosting Strategy #14

Keep junk from your lips by storing tempting foods in hard-to-reach places.

This strategy is like putting your kitchen on a diet (or your office or car, or anyplace you find yourself reaching for not-so-healthful foods). By making tempting foods less convenient to grab, you can better control your intake. Researcher Brian Wansink, PhD, of Cornell Food and Brand Lab tested this proposition. When office workers could easily reach a dish of candies that was in plain sight, they ate an average of nine pieces a day. The candy grabbing dropped to six pieces daily when the workers had to reach inside their drawers to get them and to only four pieces when the candy dish sat 6 feet from their desks. Switching up your environment like this is easier and more worth your while than relying on willpower, which fails most everyone eventually.

I didn't need to conduct a study to see this same type of result with my own patients. For example, Karen came to my office feeling as if she needed to confess. She baked four dozen cookies for her grandchildren's visit. Though she had planned to eat just a few, she ate about half of the cookies in 3 or 4 days. I asked where she had kept the cookies. Her reply: "On the kitchen counter." When she made cookies for her grandchildren's next visit, she stored them in a cabinet—not in plain sight! The cookies lasted more than just a few days, and Karen successfully limited herself to only a few.

Instead of keeping chocolate or chips in the pantry, for example, where you will see them every time you need a can of tomatoes or a box of rice, stash it in that hard-to-reach cabinet above the refrigerator. Other suggestions:

 Keep treats behind closed doors.

 Store them in opaque containers.

 Hide them behind other food.

🌿 Banish them from the house and enjoy your chips, fries, greasy chicken wings, candies, ice cream, and other splurges away from home.

Health-Boosting Strategy #15

Ease your family into lower-sodium options.

Mix one can of a "regular" product—say, canned tomatoes—with one can of its low-sodium version. Taste for salt is a learned preference, so you and your family can learn to prefer less salty foods. Just be consistent. Eventually, you will enjoy lower-sodium products without needing to mix them with higher-sodium foods. It's also okay to add a pinch of salt to low-sodium canned vegetables. Sprinkle it lightly, and you'll consume less sodium than if you used canned vegetables with added salt.

Why lower your sodium intake? A high-sodium intake is linked to high blood pressure, stroke, coronary heart disease, stomach cancer, and possibly osteoporosis and kidney stones. The American Diabetes Association recommends that everyone with diabetes limit their sodium intake to no more than 2,300 mg per day. Individuals with both diabetes and high blood pressure may or may not need to restrict their sodium intake further. The recommendations in the *Dietary Guidelines for Americans* are a bit more stringent. They say that all African Americans; people with high blood pressure, diabetes, or chronic kidney disease; and everyone aged 51 years and older should cut their sodium intake to 1,500 mg per day. The rest of the population should cap their sodium intake at 2,300 mg per day. Most Americans, however, consume significantly more than even the higher number, with an average intake of 3,400 mg daily. So regardless of which guidelines you follow, chances are better than good that you need to cut back.

Health-Boosting Strategy #16

Pre-portion hard-to-resist sweets and snacks.

If it's hard for you to eat just two cookies or a single serving of crackers, pre-portion them when you first open the package or when you arrive home from the supermarket. Decide what an appropriate portion is for you, and place that amount into a dozen or so small plastic bags or other containers. Put all of the baggies back into the original package, so that when it's time for a treat, you won't need willpower to take just a small serving.

I do this with leftover cake too. It's way too easy to eat a little bit more and then a little bit more. If you're like I am, you want to take just a sliver, but then the cake needs evening out. And the process just keeps on going. Now I slice up the whole cake, wrap each piece in wax paper, seal them all in a freezer bag or plastic container, and put the whole shebang into the freezer. A single piece defrosts quickly. This works well too for unexpected company. I take out one piece for each person. No fuss, no mess, no overindulging.

Health-Boosting Strategy #17

Rethink the meaning of value.

If your definition of *value* includes eating everything that you've paid for or everything that was given to you, I challenge you to rethink it. Many of my patients tell me that they feel compelled to fill an extra plate at a buffet or eat their full serving in a restaurant or all of the food at the kitchen table—no matter how full they are—because they simply cannot waste food. They need to get their money's worth. They may tell me that their parents grew up in the Depression and scolded them if they didn't eat everything on their plates, or they may describe having been poor college students wondering if they'd have enough money next week to buy groceries. Despite the impression made by these past experiences, overeating is not good, and eating everything on your plate doesn't help "starving children in Africa."

Value is not just about money. There is nutritional value, health value, and the pleasure value you get from taste and satisfaction. Nearly everyone cares about taste and satisfaction. If you are reading this book, you must also value nutrition and health.

If you've eaten enough food, there are three things that you can do with the uneaten portion:

1. Wrap it up for another meal, which will save you both time and money tomorrow.

2. Throw it away, because if you eat what your body does not need, the food is wasted anyway.

3. Eat it. In doing so, you ignore your body's hunger and fullness cues, overfeed yourself, and you still fail to save even a dime.

When faced with extra food, consider the harm to you from overnutrition and the value in eating just the right amount.

Health-Boosting Strategy #18
Use cues to help you stop eating.

It's not so easy to be aware of the amount of food we're eating. When we eat chips from a bag, for example, it's impossible to know if we've consumed a single serving, two servings, or even more. But if you put a handful of chips into a dish, you know when they're gone that you've eaten a handful. Eating behavior expert Brian Wansink, PhD, author of *Slim by Design: Mindless Eating Solutions for Everyday Life*, studied whether college graduate students who were free to eat unlimited chicken wings would eat less if the bones from the wings were left on the table. Indeed they did. They ate 27% less than those whose bones were removed from the table. This suggests that seeing the bones pile up kept the students aware of the amount they were consuming. A separate study conducted by different researchers found that people ate fewer pistachios when the shells were left in view than when they were removed.

Eating while multitasking or otherwise distracted isn't desirable, but we do it sometimes anyway. We can help ourselves keep track of the amount of food we eat by giving ourselves visual reminders such as those described above. Leave wrappers, popsicle sticks, shells, bones, and other food remnants on the table when eating.

Similarly, make it a house rule to eat only from a dish—and it has to be your own dish! No swiping food from other people's plates. Busy, overworked people tend to grab a bite of something here and a handful of something there. Moms especially tend to eat from their children's plates. Eating this way is less satisfying, and you can't tell how much you've consumed.

Health-Boosting Strategy #19

Reverse portions. Eat less by eating more.

Sometimes the easiest and most healthful way to eat less is to eat more—more of the low-calorie, high-nutrition, filling foods. These are the same foods that nutrition and health experts are always pushing—fruits, vegetables, and more vegetables. With this strategy, you get a double whammy of health benefits. Not only are fruits and vegetables disease-fighting foods, they fill the stomach adequately to make smaller portions of higher-calorie foods big enough. If you eat strawberry shortcake or frozen yogurt topped with fresh fruit, for example, reverse the portions to consume fewer calories and less added sugars and unhealthful fats. Next time, crumble a few bites of cake over a bowl of strawberries, or top a bowl of fruit with a dollop of frozen yogurt.

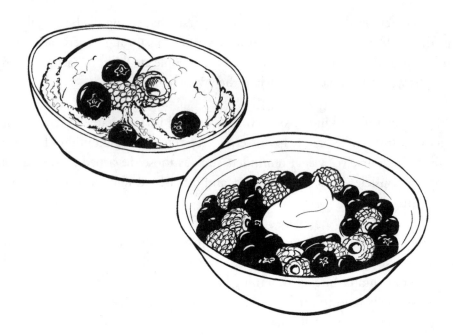

- Bowl of frozen yogurt (1 cup) topped with a sprinkling of fresh berries (1/4 cup): Calories: 242, Total Carbohydrate: 38g, Dietary Fiber: 0.8g.

- Same-size bowl filled with berries (1 cup) and topped with a large spoonful of frozen yogurt (1/4 cup): Calories: 110, Total Carbohydrate: 22g, Dietary Fiber: 3.3g. This dish saves you 132 calories.

Reverse portions on your dinner plate by doubling (even tripling) your nonstarchy veggies and shrinking your meat and starch portions by 10–30% each. At lunch, build your sandwich with a slice or two less of meat and cheese but with a double stack of vegetables. When cooking, create a rice pilaf with half rice and half vegetables instead of the traditional mere sprinkling of vegetables. You can use this strategy in soups, stews, lasagna, tuna noodle casserole, and other dishes. Only your imagination limits you, so have fun in the kitchen.

What can you expect? You will save at least a few and as many as a couple hundred calories each time you reverse portions this way. Keep it up, and you will see the pounds drop as you boost your health and reduce your risk for heart disease and other chronic health problems. You can eat the same amount of food—or even more—for fewer calories. You won't be tortured by hunger when trimming calories, counting carbs, or shaving saturated fat. Even without weight loss, many people discover that they have more energy and that their cholesterol and blood pressure levels have improved.

℣ Get It Fast Tips

℣ Keep frozen berries on hand to enjoy with a spoonful of frozen yogurt or ice cream.

℣ After defrosting frozen butternut squash purée, add to macaroni and cheese.

℣ Add prechopped carrots, celery, and onion (sold together as mirepoix) to homemade or store-bought potato salad.

℣ Fill a pita pocket with packaged broccoli slaw mix before adding tuna salad or other filling.

℣ Sneak ready-to-use shredded carrots between layers in your favorite lasagna.

℣ See Health-Boosting Strategy #3 for many similar suggestions.

Health-Boosting Strategy #20

Let your dishes control your portions.

My patient Cynthia stores leftovers and packs her lunch in portion-controlled containers from Fit & Fresh. Like measuring cups, her plastic containers are marked for volume, so she can serve herself just the amount she wants. There are lots of portion-control dishes and containers on the market these days. And they make good sense. Reining in portions of high-calorie foods is a smart strategy for weight control. Don't waste your time relying on willpower. Instead, put time and energy into strategies like this one. You'll find portion-control products in department stores, discount stores, and on the Internet.

Some have quite innovative designs that discreetly indicate where to place your portion of starch, vegetable, and meat. These are just a few sources for portion-control ware:

- Fit & Fresh (fit-fresh.com)

- Portion-Measuring Bowl Set from the American Diabetes Association (shopdiabetes.org)

- Precise Portions (preciseportions.com)

- Slimware (slimware.com)

- Wine-Trax (wine-trax.com)

You don't have to purchase all new dishes to make use of this trick. Simply measure the amount of food or beverage that your bowls and glasses can hold by filling them with water and then pouring the water into measuring cups. Pick small bowls for sweets and large bowls for salads. To limit ice cream to a 1/2-cup serving, choose a designated ice cream bowl that holds only about 1/2 cup. Designate a 1-cup bowl for cereal and hearty soups, and a 2-cup bowl for a brothy vegetable soup. As a diehard chocolate fanatic and a person too overworked and overwhelmed to worry constantly about portions, I pour dark chocolate chips into an attractive 1-ounce shot glass and savor one chip at a time.

Eating from a small plate is another smart trick. Choose a 9-inch plate instead of a typical 11-inch dinner plate, and you will both serve yourself less food and eat significantly less food, according to expert Brian Wansink, PhD. You might think this simple trick won't work, but Dr. Wansink has found that even people who are certain they are not influenced by plate size really are. You can learn more at mindlesseating.org.

Health-Boosting Strategy #21

Cook with moist heat and use other simple tactics to limit AGEs.

In case you don't know what AGEs are, advanced glycation end products are a group of compounds in our foods that may cause oxidation and inflammation and may be partly responsible for heart disease, some complications of diabetes, and other health problems. They're not a new problem, but they are only recently being studied and understood. The good news is that by using certain cooking methods over others, we can greatly reduce the amount of AGEs we consume.

AGEs are produced when sugars combine with protein, fat, or other components of your food. You see them on the darkened surface of fried chicken or a broiled steak. They give the cooked food flavor and aroma too. AGEs are naturally present in some foods, manufacturers add them to other foods, and cooking methods add even more. Large servings of meat and high-fat foods are major contributors to our AGE consumption, especially when such foods are cooked at high temperatures without liquids. Though diet is a major source, AGEs also form in the body, especially if blood glucose is elevated—just one more reason to pay careful attention to your blood glucose if you have diabetes.

Researchers have found that individuals who restrict their AGE consumption show reduced levels of inflammation and oxidative stress. One small study in a 2011 issue of *Diabetes Care* even showed improved insulin sensitivity among people with type 2 diabetes when they consumed less AGEs. Here's how to reduce your AGE intake:

✔ COOK WITH MOISTURE. Instead of grilling, browning, roasting, and frying, cook by steaming, stewing, poaching, and braising.

✔ COOK SLOW AND LOW. Use your slow cooker often and without browning the meat first.

- **COOK WITH ACIDS.** Marinate meats before grilling or broiling. Cook with vinegar, citrus juice, tomato juice, and other acidic foods to help prevent the formation of AGEs when cooking at high temperatures.

- **GRILL CORN, VEGETABLES, AND FRUIT MORE THAN BURGERS, STEAK, FISH, AND CHICKEN.** Grilling increases the AGEs of these foods too, but by a tiny amount compared with grilling high-protein and high-fat foods.

- **THINK LEAN.** High-fat foods contain more AGEs, so use lean meats, more egg whites than yolks, and reduced-fat cheeses.

- **THINK SMALL WHEN IT COMES TO MEAT.** Meats are a major source of AGEs, so don't fill your plate with them. Instead, fill your plate with lots of vegetables, which like fruits and grains are relatively low in AGEs.

- **FAVOR WHOLE FOODS OVER HIGHLY PROCESSED FOODS.** When manufacturers process grains into crispy, crunchy, fatty snack foods, their AGE content jumps.

Health-Boosting Strategy #22

Trade red meat in for other protein-rich foods.

You don't have to entirely give up steaks or hamburgers or any favorite food, but it is wise to limit your intake of red meat, which includes beef, pork, and lamb. Even though pork isn't as red as beef and lamb, for health purposes it is red meat.

According to the American Institute for Cancer Research, eating more than 18 ounces of red meat weekly increases the risk of colorectal cancer, the third most common and the third most deadly cancer in the U.S. The reasons for the association aren't clear, but red meat does contain compounds known to damage the lining of the colon. Additionally, cooking meat at high temperatures produces compounds that are harmful to health (see Health-Boosting Strategy

#21). Red meat appears to harm the heart as well. In a study that followed more than 84,000 women for 26 years, researchers found that women who ate two servings of red meat daily compared with women who ate a half serving per day had a 30% higher risk of developing coronary heart disease. Eating poultry, fish, or nuts in place of one serving of red meat daily reduced the risk of coronary heart disease by 19–30%. Even diabetes has been linked to red meat intake. Red meat is frequently rich in the unhealthy saturated fats and cholesterol, but even lean red meats are associated with health risks.

BOTTOM LINE
Eat beef, pork, and lamb only now and then. When you do, choose the leanest varieties.

✌ Get It Fast Tips

Next time you eat steak, keep your portion to no more than 4 ounces. Trade in a ham sandwich for a chicken, turkey, tuna salad, or almond butter sandwich. Instead of eating a hamburger, try a veggie burger. Or cook up salmon or turkey burgers. Buy them premade and keep them in your freezer or quickly make your own. Keep 90% (or higher) lean ground turkey in your freezer and a couple of cans of salmon in your pantry. A quick search on the Internet turns up a variety of recipes for salmon burgers. You probably have the ingredients on hand—typically salmon, onion, light mayonnaise, eggs or egg whites, herbs, and spices.

Health-Boosting Strategy #23

Squelch unhealthful snacking with a prewritten list.

Unless you're very active, your snacks should range from about 100 to 250 calories each. Athletes and very active people, however, may need several larger snacks each day. If you don't want to eat between meals and don't need snacks to control hunger, skip them and eat just three balanced meals. If you choose to snack, select foods that you don't eat enough of at meals—very likely fruits and vegetables. Many of my patients write a list of five to eight snacks that they both enjoy and can keep on hand. The list frees them from the mental energy of weighing options every time they want a snack, and it helps them to make the better choice automatically. I use a simple sheet like the one on page 87 for my patients. Include on your list the portion size that is appropriate for you. If you count calories or carbs, include these numbers next to the snack.

Here are a few snack ideas to get you started:

- any fresh, frozen, or canned fruit without added sugar

- low-fat cottage cheese with whole-grain crackers such as Triscuit Thin Crisps

- raw veggies dipped into low-fat cottage cheese mixed with salsa

- Greek yogurt with fresh or frozen berries

- an ounce of any nut (about 1/4 cup), such as walnuts, almonds, pistachios, and peanuts

- half a peanut butter or almond butter sandwich, or nut butter on whole-grain crackers. I do not mean the premade peanut butter crackers available in vending machines. These tend not to have the same nutritional value.

- reduced-fat cheese with raw veggies and grapes

- hummus and raw vegetables in a whole-wheat pita pocket

- hard-boiled egg with vegetables, fruit, or whole-grain crackers

- popcorn

- small portion of last night's leftovers

Snack Choices

_____   _____

_____   _____

_____   _____

_____   _____

_____   _____

_____   _____

_____   _____

_____   _____

_____   _____

_____   _____

_____   _____

_____   _____

_____   _____

_____   _____

_____   _____

_____   _____

Health-Boosting Strategy #24

Plan for emergencies with emergency foods.

Without both a plan and a backup plan, junk food and high-calorie fast food fare might be what's on the menu. I always have what I call emergency foods on hand as Plan B—a solution for those times when my original plan fails. What foods can you keep at work to substitute for the packed lunch that you accidentally left sitting on the kitchen counter at home? What should you have on hand if your planned snack didn't satisfy, and what do you do if you're stuck late at a meeting or in heavy traffic when your stomach is grumbling loudly?

Keep some of these emergency foods at work and at home, in the car or your purse, in your gym bag, and anyplace you might find yourself unexpectedly hungry and without appropriate food choices. Add your own ideas too.

- FROZEN OR SHELF-STABLE MEAL. See Chapter 1 for suggestions and criteria for picking one.

- MEAL REPLACEMENT. Choose a beverage or nutrition bar with at least 10 grams of protein and at most 3 grams of saturated fat. It should have no trans fat. Check out Orgain Organic Nutritional Shake (orgain.com). Many shakes and bars are very low in fiber; if yours doesn't contain at least 5 grams of fiber, have it with a piece of fruit or a vegetable, if possible. If you have diabetes, pay attention to the amount of carbohydrates in your meal replacement. Stick to the amount that is appropriate for you.

- POUCHES OF READY-TO-EAT TUNA OR SALMON.

- ANY TYPE OF NUT IN 1-OUNCE SERVINGS, TYPICALLY ABOUT 1/4 CUP. Either buy single-serving packages or premeasure them into baggies or an old tin that held breath mints. I keep two tins in my purse—one filled with nuts and the other a combination of nuts and dried fruit.

✌ ANY UNSWEETENED DRIED FRUIT. Sunsweet® sells individually wrapped prunes as well as small packages of prunes that provide 60 calories and apricots that provide 70 calories. Sun-Maid and other brands sell small packages of raisins.

✌ SINGLE-SERVING PACKETS OF PEANUT BUTTER OR ALMOND BUTTER OR A LARGER CONTAINER FOR THE OFFICE. Eat it with whole-grain crackers or pretzels.

✌ LOW-FAT YOGURT OR COTTAGE CHEESE FOR YOUR OFFICE REFRIGERATOR.

✌ SMALL CANS OF TOMATO OR VEGETABLE JUICE LIKE V8.

✌ SNACK BARS MADE OF WHOLE GRAINS OR OTHER WHOLESOME INGREDIENTS. Among others, look for Kashi® granola bars and Larabars.

If you're the type to nibble on snacks just because they are nearby, take an extra step now to avoid testing your willpower later. Put your emergency food for work in a brown paper bag, label it, and staple it closed. Keep emergency snacks for the car in the backseat.

BONUS TIPS

Having a Plan C is also a smart idea. Make a list of suitable takeout choices, so you'll know your best options before you're ready to order. Use the restaurant's online nutrition information as well as online nutrition databases such as SuperTracker.usda.gov and MyFoodAdvisor.com. Keep your lists on index cards or in your smartphone. You might prefer separate lists for each restaurant you visit. If you are a carb counter for diabetes control or a calorie counter for weight control, identify the carbohydrates or calories in your choices.

Health-Boosting Strategy #25

Sit down, slow down, and savor every bite.

I know this request is a tough one for people with hectic lives. You rush through your meals precisely because you are busy and overworked. But the practice of paying full attention to your food is important enough that I urge you to find time for it—at least for most of your meals and snacks. Planning your meals in advance, keeping your pantry properly stocked, and having emergency food on hand (see Health-Boosting Strategy #24) are important topics discussed elsewhere in this book. By using these strategies, you will find that you can make time to eat sitting down (not in the car) while noticing and enjoying every bite.

Why do I think this matters so much? There is a lot of mindless eating and rapid eating going on, and they result in both excess calories and less pleasure. Have you ever been so rushed to eat or so overhungry that you ate a large amount of food very quickly and didn't feel full until several minutes later? And by then you were overfull? Most of us have experienced this at least a few times. When we eat so fast, we often don't get the signals that we've had enough until we've overeaten. Think back to those times. Were they even pleasurable? Probably not.

Some benefits to sitting down, slowing down, and savoring every bite:

💈 You will be physically satisfied with less food.

💈 You will be psychologically satisfied with less food.

💈 You will enjoy your meals and snacks more.

💈 You will feel less harried.

💈 You may experience less heartburn and other gastrointestinal upset.

If you're still not convinced that it's worth making time to be fully engaged with your food, try this experiment. It's eye-opening. Take two identical pieces or bites of a favorite candy. I typically use Hershey's Kisses, but use anything that you like very much. Eat one very fast, as if you were in a speed-eating contest. Then place the second one in your mouth and swirl it around, noticing its taste and texture. Bite into it and swirl it around some more. Finish it slowly, all the while noticing the taste and how it feels in your mouth. When you are done, think about the two experiences and the benefits of eating slowly, noticing your food, and savoring every bite.

Get started on this practice by picking as few as four meals this week to eat slowly and mindfully. Before getting up from the table, reflect on the experience. At the end of the week, evaluate the pleasure and overall experience of those meals compared to eating when you were not fully engaged. I think you will see that it's much better to make eating the event instead of something we do while multitasking.

BONUS TIP FOR RESTAURANT EATING

Be the slowest eater at the table. Other people influence what we eat, how much we eat, and how quickly we eat it. Research has shown that you're likely to eat more when dining with friendly people. Interestingly, the more people in the group, the larger the meal becomes. We even copy the speed at which others eat. And the faster we eat, the more we eat. Remember that Brian Wansink has studied the effects of environmental factors on eating behaviors, and his research shows that even people who strongly believe that they are not influenced by such things really are (see Health-Boosting Strategy #20).

I try to stay on my toes to limit how others affect what and how I eat. My trick is to have a contest that only I know about. I try to be the slowest eater at the table—the last to pick up my fork and the one to always have the most food left on the plate.

Chapter 5:
EAT BETTER

Healthful eating is about more than eating this and limiting that. In this chapter, you'll learn to preserve nutrients, balance your meals, make meals enjoyable, cultivate a constructive attitude, and more.

Health-Boosting Strategy #26

Chop garlic 10 minutes early.

Make this the first step of your recipe. Why? Chopping or crushing garlic activates its natural disease-fighting phytochemicals, but heat instantly deactivates those same compounds. Allowing the chopped garlic to sit at room temperature for as little as 10 minutes before cooking helps retain most of its health-promoting properties.

So what can garlic do for your health? According to the American Institute for Cancer Research, garlic probably protects against colorectal cancer. Additionally, garlic is a member of the allium family of vegetables, which also includes onions, leeks, and chives. Eating allium vegetables is linked to a lower risk of stomach cancer. Garlic is also being studied for possible roles in the prevention of heart disease.

You can use crushed raw garlic to make a quick vinaigrette with olive oil, lemon juice, and fresh herbs such as cilantro or basil.

Health-Boosting Strategy #27

Balance your meals for sustained energy and good nutrition.

Now and then, people tell me—almost in a boastful way—that they ate only vegetables for dinner the night before. Sure, I'm happy they ate lots of vegetables, but that's not a balanced meal any more than if they ate only steak or fish, or nothing but peanuts and pineapple. Eating balanced meals assures that you're getting balanced nutrition. It also helps you to feel full and maintain energy to work on whatever tasks are ahead of you. Frequently, when people complain to me about being terribly hungry shortly after lunch or breakfast, or hitting the afternoon slump barely after noon, I find that the culprit is a skimpy or unbalanced meal.

Eat at least three food groups at each meal and in large enough portions that you aren't famished an hour or two later. Each meal should include good sources of fiber, protein, and healthy fats. Here are examples to help you plan your meals:

✌ Breakfast

- whole-wheat toast with peanut butter and banana, an egg, and a glass of milk or soymilk

- oatmeal, diced apple, walnuts, milk or soymilk, and a hard-boiled egg

- cottage cheese, raisins, and muesli

- See Health-Boosting Strategy #28 for more tips.

✌ Lunch/Dinner

- black bean soup, whole-grain crackers, Greek yogurt mixed with fresh berries and sliced almonds

- tuna salad made with light mayonnaise, whole-wheat pita bread, lettuce, tomato, and a pear on the side

- salad of leftover rice or quinoa tossed with baby spinach, diced bell peppers, cherry tomatoes, steamed shrimp or deli-sliced turkey, and Italian vinaigrette; apple on the side

Health-Boosting Strategy #28

Spread your protein out over the day.

Until recently, I didn't worry about my patients' protein intake. Nearly everyone eats an adequate amount over the course of the day. But recent research suggests that the distribution of the protein is even more important than the total amount of protein consumed. I've noticed that the majority of my patients eat very little protein at breakfast, a little bit more at lunch, and quite a lot at dinner. These days, I ask them to better spread their protein out over their three meals. Here's why:

FOR WEIGHT CONTROL: Eating protein-rich foods helps control hunger, and inadequate protein appears to increase the desire to eat.

FOR BODY COMPOSITION: Protein stimulates muscle synthesis, and it takes about 30 grams of protein for maximal stimulation. As we age, we tend to lose muscle mass—about 3–8% per decade after age 30. By eating adequate protein over the day, muscle synthesis is stimulated more often. Additionally, when we cut calories to lose weight, we drop more than body fat. Initially, we lose water weight, but we also lose muscle mass. When protein intake is greater, we lose more body fat and less muscle mass. With proper diet and strength-training exercises, it's even possible to gain muscle mass while losing body fat.

BOTTOM LINE
Eat moderate amounts of lean protein (about 25–30 grams) at each of your three meals. More is not better, and less probably does not stimulate muscle

synthesis adequately or suitably control hunger. Whenever possible, plan your physical activity close in time to your protein intake.

❧ Get It Fast Tips

For many people it's harder to consume adequate protein at breakfast than at other meals. Nearly everyone is time-crunched first thing in the morning. Keep Greek yogurt (higher in protein than traditional yogurt), low-fat cottage cheese, hard-boiled eggs, and nontraditional choices such as canned beans, deli-sliced turkey, and cans of tuna on hand. Here are a few breakfast meal ideas to get you started:

❧ 1 cup plain or vanilla Greek yogurt, fruit, 1/2 cup Post Grape-Nuts or Kashi® GoLean® cereal

❧ 1 cup 2% cottage cheese, fruit, almonds or walnuts

❧ veggie omelet with egg substitute or 1 egg and 2 egg whites, 1 cup nonfat or 1% milk, 1 slice whole-wheat bread

❧ turkey sandwich (2 slices whole-grain bread, 2 1/2 ounces turkey, lettuce, tomato)

❧ 1 cup black beans with salsa and reduced-fat Cheddar cheese, wrapped in flour tortilla

❧ smoothie of 1 cup soymilk, banana, 3 tablespoons hemp seeds, 2 tablespoons peanut butter

Health-Boosting Strategy #29

Use the glycemic index as an adjunct to other meal-planning techniques.

Patients, especially those with diabetes, often ask me about the glycemic index (GI). They've heard about it and want to try it. I'm okay with that for fine-tuning their food choices, but they should use other meal-planning strategies too.

The GI ranks carbohydrate-containing foods from 0 to 100, indicating how a single food in a portion containing 50 grams of carbohydrate is expected to affect blood glucose. The greater the number, the greater the expected effect. You can find the GI of various foods at glycemicindex.com.

When people with diabetes combine the GI with other methods of diabetes meal planning—such as carbohydrate counting—their average blood glucose level improves. Studies suggest that using the GI lowers A1C, a measure of long-term blood glucose control, by 0.2–0.5 percentage points, a small but meaningful amount. Studies also suggest that low-GI diets may protect against endometrial cancer, heart disease, and other health problems. Research is conflicting, however, particularly because studies do not control for the amount of fiber in various diets, making it unclear if the fiber content or the glycemic index of the diet is responsible for the findings.

You can run into nutritional trouble if you base your food choices solely on the GI. Grapes are clearly a more nutritious snack than ice cream, but ice cream has the lower GI score. Potatoes, whole-wheat bread, and bananas, for example, all have relatively high GI scores, but they are wholesome foods that provide needed nutrients. The GI also changes depending on what else is eaten at the meal and how the food is prepared. Portion size is also critically important to your health and blood glucose values, but not to a GI score. The GI is based on a serving size that contains 50 grams of digestible carbohydrate, so the GI of a small piece of cake is the same as the GI of a large piece of cake. The large piece, though, will have a greater effect on blood glucose. In one sitting, we rarely eat food in portions containing exactly 50 grams of carbohydrate—as, for example, in 1 1/2 pounds of carrots or 9 cups of cherry tomatoes!

GLYCEMIC LOAD. The glycemic load (GL) reflects both the GI and the portion size. Thus, the GL varies with the amount of food you consume.
Foods with a low GL: ≤10
Foods with a high GL: ≥20

Below is the simple formula for calculating the GL and examples using two portions of watermelon. You must know both the GI of the food and the amount of carbohydrates in your portion. Find the GI at glycemicindex.com, and use food labels, online nutrition databases (such as MyFoodAdvisor™ and the USDA National Nutrient Database), and carb-counting books to learn the amount of carbohydrates in your portion.

GL Formula:

❧ Glycemic Load = (GI × grams of carbohydrate eaten)/100
Watermelon: GI = 72

Example #1: 1-cup serving of melon balls contains 12 grams carbohydrate

❧ GL = (72 × 12)/100 = **8.6**
In this example, you can see that eating 1 cup of watermelon has a low GL. But what if you ate a very large portion of watermelon? In the next example, the GL is quite large.

Example #2: 4-cup serving of melon balls contains 48 grams carbohydrate

❧ GL = (72 × 48)/100 = **34.6**

These examples illustrate how complicated it is to use the GI and the GL, and why I want my patients to first learn other techniques to choose their foods. The greatest benefit to using the GI/GL comes when making choices between similar foods. For example, a baked potato with skin has lower scores than a baked potato without the skin, and an underripe banana has lower scores than a ripe banana. Al dente spaghetti is lower than well-cooked spaghetti, and an orange is lower than orange juice. If the GI and GL interest you, visit the University of Sydney website at glycemicindex.com, where you can search the GI of various foods.

Health-Boosting Strategy #30

Create a cheat sheet.

If you're just starting to pay attention to calories or carbs or generally want to boost your knowledge about the amounts in your favorite foods or recipes, use a chart like the one here. Start by listing your favorite foods or recipes in the first column. As you buy or eat the food or prepare the recipe, fill in the rest of the columns. Soon you'll have an individualized cheat sheet, making calorie or carb counting much simpler, faster, and more accurate.

FOOD	SERVING SIZE	CALORIES/ CARBOHYDRATE IN 1 SERVING	MY USUAL PORTION	CALORIES/ CARBOHYDRATE IN MY PORTION
Bagel chips	3/4 cup	180 calories/ 22 grams carbohydrate	1/2 cup	120 calories/ 15 grams carbohydrate

Health-Boosting Strategy #31

Give up the all-or-nothing approach.

This whole book is based on the premise that small changes add up to big results over time. Unfortunately, messages from the media tell us to strive for perfection, to never eat "bad" foods, and to feel decadent or guilty when we do. Often, when I meet new patients, they describe dinner the night before as a last hurrah of sorts. They are so certain I will require them to give up their favorite foods that they try to cram in as many as possible the night before their new diet starts. This is never a smart idea.

When people who embrace an all-or-nothing diet stray from their list of diet rules once, they then tend to stray even more. They go through another last hurrah for a meal or two, or a day or two or longer, until they go back on their diet—often on a Monday. At best, this all-or-nothing approach keeps things the same. At worst, it leads to weight gain, high cholesterol levels, greater insulin resistance, and other problems, including lowered self-esteem.

If you routinely start your diet over, make or try to follow long lists of diet rules, feel deprived when trying to lose weight or better your health, or feel guilty if you eat a "bad" food, you will benefit from a little moderation. I favor the 90-10 rule or the 80-20 rule, or even the 75-25 rule. However you choose to label it, it simply means that if most of the time—say 80% of the time—you eat well, then it's all right to relax the other times. Relax doesn't mean gorge, but it does mean that you might enjoy a small piece of birthday cake or some fried foods periodically. The best part is that you can really enjoy them. There's no guilt! Why should there be any guilt if you usually make nutritious choices? And even if you relaxed too much and ate too much birthday cake, for example, it's still not a big deal as long as the overindulgence ends right there and you don't plan your next last hurrah.

This concept of moderation is scary to people who find safety in diet rules. Following rules means that you don't have to make decisions or use your own judgment. Some people think that they can't trust themselves to make decisions. But strict diets don't work in the long run. If you've lost weight before on a strict diet only to gain it all back, then you already know that strict diets eventually fail. It is not because you are a failure; it is because you chose an unrealistic plan. There is room for moderation, but there is no room for either very strict diet rules or the other extreme of eating anything and everything. One treat or dietary indiscretion mustn't lead to more dietary indiscretions.

Embracing moderation is liberating because it shows you that eating a treat either by choice or because of poor judgment doesn't alter the bigger picture. Planning is important, but so is flexibility. Health-Boosting Strategy #32 builds on this concept.

Health-Boosting Strategy #32

Give yourself a treat allowance.

This strategy allows you to eat anything you want. I love chocolate—really, really love it. Unfortunately, it's everywhere—in the checkout aisle of the grocery store, on nearly every receptionist's desk, at gatherings of friends and coworkers. Without my allowance strategy, I would likely eat way more chocolate than I do.

What if you treated food the way you treat money? Say you had a gift card for $100, or even $1,000, to your favorite clothing or small electronics store. You could go into that store and walk out with anything you wanted. But you could not walk out with everything you wanted because you would soon use up the money on your gift card. The same is true for food. You can have anything you want (unless you are allergic or intolerant) but not everything you want or in the amount you want and still have a healthful diet. By giving yourself a treat allowance, you have permission to have treats in a controlled amount. My daily treat allowance is up to 150 dessert calories (I don't care for fried foods or other types of treats, so typically all of my allowance goes to dessert— chocolate specifically). If you have diabetes, you might want to give yourself a treat allowance in calories and carbohydrates. Perhaps your dessert will cap at 15 grams of carbohydrates and 150 calories. This is just an example; choose what works for you and your health goals.

Now take the money analogy one step further. You need to budget your money to meet your financial goals and obligations: paying rent or mortgage, electricity, buying gas for your car. After you've paid for all of your necessities, you can spend a portion of what's left on movies, vacations, jewelry, and other fun things. Similarly, you need to budget your calories to meet your weight and health goals. Eating fruits and vegetables, whole grains, and other nutrient-dense foods comes first. If your diet is quite good, you can spend the calories, carbs, saturated fats, or whatever is left in your budget on your favorite splurges.

Having my allowance keeps me from fighting with myself over whether I should or shouldn't eat dessert. It's simply built into my balanced diet plan. The mental energy I've saved can be used to build other skills and to be creative in other areas of my life.

Health-Boosting Strategy #33

Personalize your health plan.

Talk about a time-waster! In my two decades of counseling patients for healthy eating, diabetes management, and weight loss, I haven't seen anything suck up energy and time as much as following one fad after another or looking for that one plan that finally works. Weight loss is hard. If it were easy, there would be no overweight people! Eating healthfully when we are busy with our overscheduled lives and constantly faced with large portions of high-calorie foods is hard. Instead of hunting for that perfect diet plan, accept that you must do the difficult work in order to succeed. Interestingly, once people do realize this, an enormous weight is lifted from them. They eat with more confidence and without guilt. And the best part is that they finally do reach their health goals—and with a plan to maintain their healthy eating habits.

If you have bounced around from diet plan to diet plan, followed strict and arbitrary rules only to completely give them up a short time later, make a vow now to work toward smarter, better eating that fits your life and your goals. On your own or with the guidance of a registered dietitian nutritionist (RD or RDN), review your current eating habits and identify areas for improvement. Pick one or even a few dietary changes. They should be neither so hard that you are bound to fail nor so easy that you get nothing from them. Write these dietary goals down. Are they so specific that you—or even a stranger who reads them—will know exactly what you are going to do? If not, rewrite them.

Examples of vague goals:

❦ I'll eat better.

❦ I'll eat less junk food.

❦ I won't drink so much soda.

Some specific goals:

❦ I'll eat two servings of fruit and at least 1 1/2 cups of nonstarchy vegetables every weekday.

❦ I'll allow myself one dessert on each of 3 days this week, and each dessert will have no more than 250 calories.

❦ Instead of drinking soda with lunch, I'll have flavored water or unsweetened iced tea every day this week.

When you've mastered these goals, pick a few more, then a few more, and so on. Give up the notion that there is a best plan or an easy plan. Your best plan is the one you can live with, allows you some flexibility, and gets you to your goals—even if it takes longer than you'd like.

HINT: Visit the website for the Academy of Nutrition and Dietetics (eatright. org) to find a registered dietitian nutritionist in your area. Click on Find a Registered Dietitian in the upper right-hand corner. You will be directed to enter your zip code.

Health-Boosting Strategy #34

Replace unhealthy saturated and trans fats with unsaturated fats.

Let's try to forget the 1980s when fat was bad and fat-free cookies were all the rage. Today we know that the type of fat matters more than the quantity of fat. And cookies—whether fat-free, made with whole grains, or fortified with vitamins and fiber—are still cookies and never health food. Besides, having some fat with each of your meals helps you to absorb fat-soluble vitamins and disease-fighting phytochemicals.

Unsaturated fats are the ones to choose. Omega-9 fatty acids are monounsaturated fats. Polyunsaturated fats include both omega-6 and omega-3 fatty acids. Only a few years ago, researchers and health professionals were concerned that omega-6 fatty acids might be harmful to the heart. The American Heart Association and the World Health Organization have recently reported that this is not a concern. When it comes to fat, your best bet is to replace unhealthy saturated and trans fats with unsaturated fats. The switch will improve both cholesterol levels and insulin resistance.

As a rule of thumb, saturated fats are hard at room temperature. They include butter, lard, bacon grease, and beef fat. Milk fat and the tropical oils (coconut, palm, and palm kernel) are also largely saturated. If you tried to eat no saturated fatty acids, you'd soon go hungry because you would have few food choices. Fats are combinations of fatty acids, so even salmon and olive and canola oils, which are good sources of healthy fats, contain some saturated fatty acids. Most people should aim for no more than about 10–20 grams of saturated fats per day, though this amount will vary depending on an individual's calorie needs and health status.

Trans fats largely come from partially hydrogenated oils. You'll find them in processed foods such as crackers, snack cakes, and packaged meals. Read labels carefully to identify traces of trans fats. If you see *partially hydrogenated oil,* you know that there are at least traces of trans fat present, even if the label says No Trans Fat. The law permits the label to read zero if there is less than 0.5 grams trans fat per serving. Try to avoid trans fats as much as possible. Even those traces add up.

Swap the unhealthy for the healthy:

- Eat fatty fish like salmon and tuna (see Health-Boosting Strategy #6) at least twice weekly in place of red meats, poultry with skin, pizza, and the like.

- Snack on a handful of nuts instead of sweets.

- Add creaminess to salads with chunks of avocado.

- Sprinkle nuts instead of croutons over a salad.

- When baking a cake, quick bread, and even some cookies, replace 4 tablespoons of butter with 3 tablespoons of olive or canola oil.

- Substitute all or half of the butter in your recipe with canola or olive oils.

- Trade in cheesy dressings and sauces for vinaigrettes.

- Put together a peanut butter sandwich—as quick as making a bologna sandwich and faster than picking up a pizza.

- In restaurants and at home, trade in the full-fat cheese on your sandwich for a slice of avocado.

- Choose foods with omega-3 fatty acids often: fish, canola oil, ground flaxseeds, hemp and chia seeds, walnuts, soybeans, and tofu.

Health-Boosting Strategy #35

Go halfsies.

Sometimes substituting a wholesome ingredient for one that's not-so-wholesome just plain ruins a recipe. Do you really want chocolate cake or blueberry muffins made with whole-wheat flour? If that leaves you with a plate of hard-as-rocks treats that are no treat at all, it isn't worth doing. Since healthful eating isn't an all-or-nothing activity, substitute where you can—say, 1% milk for whole milk and reduced-fat cheese for regular cheese. There's no reason to go all the way to nonfat milk and cheeses if you then don't even want to eat your meal. If your recipe doesn't tolerate any substitution, simply eat a very small portion. In many cases, however, you can mix two ingredients or cut back just a little to improve the nutrient profile of your recipe while maintaining the desired taste and texture. For example, your muffins may turn out exquisitely when prepared with a combination of white and whole-wheat flours. Try these substitutions.

Health-Boosting Strategy #36

Don't toss nutrients out in the cooking water.

To preserve vitamins, minerals, and phytochemicals in your vegetables, cook them quickly and use little water. Steaming and microwaving in a small amount of water (the key is *small*) is ideal. Boiling vegetables leaches nutrients into the water. Stir-frying and oven roasting are two more great ways to cook vegetables, but use a light hand with the oil to keep calories down if you are watching your weight. Though oven roasting uses high heat and requires fairly long cooking times, you won't lose as much of the nutrients as you would if you cooked in water. For more nutrients, keep the skins on too.

So what should you do if you really prefer boiled-until-soft veggies? Well, boiled veggies are way better than no veggies, so if boiling them helps you to

INSTEAD OF THIS	TRY THIS
Ground beef	94% lean ground beef or ground turkey
Half-and-half	Fat-free half-and-half, milk, evaporated fat-free milk
Cheese	Reduced-fat cheese
Sour cream	Reduced-fat sour cream or Greek yogurt
Cornflake crumbs	Crushed Wheaties®
Enriched white flour	Whole-wheat flour, whole-wheat pastry flour, white whole-wheat flour (these last two are softer and lighter)
Butter in baked goods	Replace 4 tablespoons of butter with 3 tablespoons of canola or olive oil.
Sugar in baking	Reduce by 1/4–1/2 or use in combination with sugar substitutes.
Bagels, sub rolls, and other large rolls	Cut the calorie and carbs by scooping out and discarding the doughy center from your rolls and bagels.
Mayonnaise	Light mayonnaise, smashed avocado, or hummus
Wine	Enjoy a wine spritzer by diluting the wine with an equal amount of seltzer or club soda.

eat lots, then stick with it. If you can reuse the boiling water in soups or stews, do that too.

Finally, don't fall for the advice to eat all of your fruits and vegetables raw. Absorption of some nutrients increases when the food is cooked. For example, cooking tomatoes (think broiled summer tomatoes, pasta sauce, and canned tomatoes) actually boosts the availability of lycopene, a phytochemical cousin to beta-carotene. Cooking softens the cell wall, making lycopene more accessible, and it changes the structure of lycopene, increasing its absorption.

BONUS TIP

Broccoli, cauliflower, cabbage, arugula, kale, mustard greens, radish, watercress, wasabi, and horseradish are cruciferous vegetables. This unique family of vegetables contains compounds that can be converted to health-shielding phytochemicals, which, among other things, may decrease inflammation and detoxify cancer-causing compounds. Excessive heat inactivates this conversion, but some heat is actually good. To maximize the health boosters in cruciferous vegetables, my friend and colleague Karen Collins, MS, RDN, CDN, nutrition consultant to the American Institute for Cancer Research, suggests using one of the following cooking methods:

- Steam for up to 4 minutes.

- Blanch in boiling water for about 30 seconds.

- When eating cruciferous vegetables that have been cooked longer, season with strong mustard or wasabi, or eat a raw crucifer such as arugula or radishes at the same meal.

If you'd like to learn more about diet for cancer prevention, take a look at Karen Collins' blog Smart Bytes® (karencollinsnutrition.com/smartbytes) and the website for the American Institute for Cancer Research (aicr.org).

BOTTOM LINE

Eat lots of cooked and raw fruits and vegetables. Any fruit and vegetable is better than no fruit and vegetable. When possible, cook vegetables in just small amounts of water.

Health-Boosting Strategy #37

Wash before eating, peeling, or cutting.

Always wash your hands in preparation for these activities, of course. But don't forget to wash your produce. Doing so—and in the proper manner—goes a long way in keeping you and your family safe from food poisoning. Bacteria in the soil or water can contaminate any produce. Even organic produce needs to be washed. Follow these guidelines:

- Use cold running water from your tap. You do not need soap or special produce rinses.

- To keep bacteria from being transferred from the outside of your produce to the inside, wash melons, oranges, cucumbers, and all other fruits and vegetables even if you plan to peel them before eating.

- Scrub cantaloupe, potatoes, and other firm fruits and vegetables with a produce brush, especially if they have textured or bumpy skins.

- Discard the outer leaves of lettuce, cabbage, and other leafy greens before washing.

- Dry washed produce with a clean cloth or paper towel.

- Don't buy bruised or damaged fruits and vegetables. If you find such produce at home, cut and discard damaged areas. That's where bacteria lurk.

- Use separate cutting boards for produce and uncooked meats.

Know that bean sprouts, alfalfa sprouts, and other sprouts are likely sources of bacteria, including *Salmonella*, *E. coli*, and *Listeria*. These bacteria cannot be washed away from sprouts. You must cook sprouts thoroughly to reduce the risk of illness. This goes for restaurant food or even sprouts you have grown yourself. Children, the elderly, pregnant women, and anyone with a weakened immune system should not eat raw or lightly cooked sprouts of any kind.

BONUS TIP
Make sure bagged salads and precut produce are refrigerated or kept on ice before buying, and put them in the refrigerator immediately once home.

Health-Boosting Strategy #38

Cook it safe, and know when to toss it out.

More than 100,000 Americans are hospitalized each year because of food poisoning. Improperly cooked foods are a major reason for it. Use a meat thermometer to know if your food is thoroughly cooked. Place the thermometer in the thickest part of the food, making sure not to touch bone, fat, or gristle. Copy the following guide for the minimum safe cooking temperature onto an index card; place it on your refrigerator or elsewhere in your kitchen or near your outdoor grill.

- ground meat: 165°F

- steak: 145°F

- pork: 145°F

- poultry: 165°F

- fin fish: 145°F

- leftovers and casseroles: 165°F

🌱 egg dishes: 160°F

Find additional information at foodsafety.gov.

Instead of having to chase down food safety information every time you have a question—or worse, risk getting sick because you didn't take the time to look it up—download the free app Is My Food Safe? for Android and Apple mobile devices. With this app, you'll find safe cooking temperatures as well as guidelines for how long you can keep certain foods like opened ketchup bottles and leftover chicken.

Health-Boosting Strategy #39

Take a minute to zap germs.

Get rid of bacteria, molds, and yeasts. Your kitchen sponge is a breeding ground and safe harbor to such illness-causing nuisances. Zap your sponge in the microwave for 1 minute or run it through your dishwasher with the drying cycle on. Scientists at the USDA Agricultural Research Service found that both of these methods killed more than 99% of the bacteria, yeast, and molds present.

What methods didn't work? Soaking the dirty sponge in a 10% chlorine bleach solution, lemon juice, and de-ionized water were all failures. Get in the habit of cleaning your sponge in the microwave or dishwasher every day or two, and replace it frequently. Your sponge should be damp when you put it into your microwave. It will get hot, so use caution taking it out.

Health-Boosting Strategy #40

Pack lunch—even when you eat at home.

I never packed a lunch for eating at home until recently, but it has been a big calorie saver and nutrient booster. I work at home on my writing and consulting projects several days a week. Working on both this book and another one distracted me from my midday hunger pangs until they were nearly out of control. After a week or so of running downstairs to hurriedly find lunch because I was in-pain hungry, I had a brilliant idea: pack lunch as if I were going to my patient office. What a difference a few minutes in the morning or the night before have made! Now, I simply walk downstairs, take my packed lunch from the refrigerator, and sit down to a balanced meal.

In general, packing or planning lunch is an important strategy for healthful eating. Tammy has been my patient for almost 4 months. She's dropped 25 pounds so far. Many things have contributed to her success, and packing lunch is one of them. In fact, Tammy packs both breakfast and lunch for work every day. Though she does still treat herself, these days it's rare for her to eat a burger and fries for lunch. Instead, on Sunday, she packs everything she needs for breakfast and lunch for the entire week. When she arrives to work on Monday morning, she's set for the next 5 days. I nearly always encourage my patients to pack lunch for work instead of relying on fast food or restaurant meals. Eating out probably costs you more calories and unhealthful fats than you realize. Even salads often tip the scales at 800 or more calories and a day's worth of saturated fat and sodium. Another advantage to eating a home-prepared lunch is that no one asks if you want fries or apple pie with that. Here are the basic rules for lunch (and any other meal):

✌ Eat enough food to keep you from getting hungry quickly.

✌ Include a mix of protein, fiber, and healthy fats. (See Health-Boosting Strategies #27 and #34.)

Gather the proper lunch accessories: a thermal lunch box, reuseable cold pack, BPA-free plastic or glass containers, and BPA-free water bottle. If you like leftovers for lunch, pack them before sitting down to dinner or immediately after eating. Plan for your lunches just as you should for your dinners. Before the week starts, buy the proper groceries. Also have on hand quick-to-grab items such as the emergency foods identified in Health-Boosting Strategy #24.

Chapter 6:
BEYOND FOOD

Good health requires so much more than good nutrition. For many people, exercise is what comes to mind next. But even that is not enough. Adequate sleep and stress management are essential too. This chapter helps you manage these areas of your well-being, guiding you to prioritize activities and problem solve whatever is holding you back.

If you are not healthy enough for exercise or are not sure, seek the advice of an exercise expert and speak to your health care provider. Start off slowly and increase your time and intensity only as you build strength, and only as you are permitted and medically able.

Health-Boosting Strategy #41
Make every step count.

Clip a pedometer to your waistband or an accelerometer on your wrist, and get moving! People who wear pedometers or other step-tracking devices tend to be more active and have lower levels of obesity and healthier blood pressure levels. Step counters are very motivating and can encourage you to park farther away from your destination, walk an extra block, play active games with your kids, dance with your friends, and find many more ways to keep moving.

When shopping for a pedometer, be certain to buy a good one. The free pedometers are rarely of use; most of them count steps for every little twist and turn, even for rocking in a chair and driving over a speed bump. A good pedometer will set you back about $30. All you really need is a step counter, but if you like fancy and techy, go for it. Some pedometers have 7-day memories, track aerobic steps, and are downloadable to your computer. Here's how to get the most out of your pedometer:

✌ Clip it on to your waistband above the center of your knee. Take exactly 100 steps. If your pedometer reads between 90 and 110 steps, you have a good pedometer and it's in the right location. If your pedometer reads outside that range, move it an inch to the right or left or to the other hip. Take 100 steps again. If it still seems inaccurate, it's not a good one and you should return it.

✌ If your weight changes and your pants become very loose or so tight that the waistband rolls down, you will not get an accurate reading. Turn the pedometer inward so the face of it touches your skin, or try placing it at the small of the back. One of these adjustments usually does the trick.

✌ Put it on when you first wake up and take it off before bed. Record your steps for motivation.

✌ If you're just getting started with walking, wear your pedometer for 3 or 4 days to determine your baseline steps. Then set a weekly step goal. For example, plan to add an average of 500–2,000 daily steps by next week and then again the following week and so on, until you reach an average of at least 10,000 steps—or whatever individualized goal you and your health care team set. Work at your own pace, and don't worry about how long it takes to reach your goal.

An accelerometer may be what you want if you don't like wearing your tracking device on your waist or if you want more functions. I use an accelerometer from Fitbit, the Flex™ Wireless Activity and Sleep Wristband. It measures my steps accurately, even when I'm walking very slowly or moving at Zumba® class. If I carry it in my pocket, it measures my steps on the elliptical cross trainer and some of my movements while biking. Flex™ also records distance covered, calories burned, hours slept, and the number of awake or restless minutes during the night. There are functions to record food intake with calories, your weight, fluid intake, and more data. You can keep track of these functions online or with a smartphone app. The Flex™ and similar accelerometers such as Jawbone UP™ and Nike+ FuelBand SE are more costly than a pedometer with a price tag of about $100–$150. If your budget allows for one, it can be very helpful in meeting your goals.

Health-Boosting Strategy #42

Strength train in less time with compound exercises.

Compound exercises like push-ups use more than one joint movement. Isolation exercises such as bicep curls use just one. You can get a full-body workout much faster by engaging multiple muscle groups at one time. This is not to say that bicep curls, hamstring curls, and other isolation exercises have no value. They do. They allow you to focus on one muscle group that may be important to your sport or may simply give additional emphasis to a well-rounded strength-training program. If you want to finish your workout faster, however, compound exercises are the way to go.

Assuming you are fit enough, you will ideally work all of your major muscle groups two or three times weekly on nonconsecutive days. They are muscles in the legs, hips, back, abdomen, chest, arms, and shoulders. Most, if healthy enough, should work their muscles to exhaustion, meaning to the point that it is difficult to continue in good form without assistance. Compound exercises include squats, lunges, shoulder press, pull-ups, push-ups, chest press, and dips. Many people—women especially—make the mistake of using weights that are too light to maintain or build strength. Additionally, many people choose cardiovascular or aerobic exercises over strength training. However, both are critically important for your good health. Regular strength training offers these benefits and more:

✌ weight control

✌ improved blood glucose control

✌ relief from arthritis pain

- increased bone density and reduced risk for fractures

- decreased risk of falling, a benefit that becomes increasingly important as we age

- improved sleep

- better mood

Learn more about strength training at these reputable websites:

- Centers for Disease Control and Prevention (CDC): http://www.cdc.gov/ physicalactivity/everyone/guidelines/adults.html#Musclestrengthening

- IDEA Health and Fitness Association: http://www.ideafit.com/exercise-library

- American Council on Exercise (ACE): http://www.acefitness.org/acefit/ exercise-library-main

If you are new to strength training, seek the advice of an expert. Always consult your health care provider before engaging in new activities.

Do It Fast Tips

If you can't fit a full-body workout into a single time slot, split up upper-body and lower-body workouts. For example, perform lower-body exercises on Mondays and Wednesdays and upper-body exercises on Tuesdays and Thursdays. You could even do an upper-body workout in the morning and a lower-body workout the same afternoon, if necessary.

Health-Boosting Strategy #43

Rev up your exercise.

Cardiovascular or aerobic exercise is like a miracle drug. It helps prevent type 2 diabetes, heart disease, stroke, osteoporosis, overweight and obesity, and several types of cancer. It boosts mood, lowers blood pressure, enhances insulin sensitivity, facilitates better sleep, leads to greater mobility and function in aging, and so, so much more. Most people know the importance of exercise, yet only 58% of adults in the U.S. are minimally physically active—defined as engaging in 30 minutes of moderate or vigorous activity three times weekly. According to the CDC, most adults should engage in *at least* 150 minutes of moderate-intensity aerobic activity (fast walking, water aerobics, doubles tennis) or 75 minutes of vigorous-intensity aerobic activity (jogging, swimming laps, singles tennis) each week. This same amount of exercise was found to help prevent or delay type 2 diabetes in high-risk people.

People have all types of reasons to skip exercise, but the one I hear the most often is "I don't have time." First, take whatever time you have. You may want to exercise for 30 minutes, but if all you have is 20 or 12 or 8 minutes, then take them. Exercise is not an all-or-nothing activity. Every minute is a plus. If you haven't yet been able to form the exercise habit, consider exercising just 5 minutes every single day. See the introduction of Part 2 for more about using tiny goals to form habits. Everyone can find a mere 5 minutes.

Assuming that you make time for aerobic exercise and that you are in good physical condition, you can maximize that time with high-intensity interval training (HIIT). This type of workout involves alternating high-intensity exercise for 30–60 seconds with lower-intensity recovery exercise for 60 seconds to several minutes. Studies show that compared to exercising at a constant speed, HIIT burns more calories, results in greater fat loss, and shows bigger improvements in cholesterol levels, blood pressure, glucose regulation, and cardiovascular fitness. Check in with your health care provider before starting this or another exercise program.

Add intervals to walking, jogging, biking, or any cardiovascular exercise machine that you use (such as a rower, treadmill, or stair-climber). After warming up at a moderate pace for several minutes, sprint (or even walk at a slightly faster pace) for 30–60 seconds or some other comfortable amount of time. Return to your easier pace for 1–5 minutes. Then do another sprint. Do several cycles as tolerated. As you improve fitness, increase the frequency or length of your high-intensity exercise or decrease the length of your recovery time.

Health-Boosting Strategy #44

Cue yourself to exercise.

In our 24/7 lifestyle, who isn't too busy, too tired, or too distracted at times to exercise? Discipline (like willpower) isn't enough, so use a few of the following techniques to make your workout plan a reality:

🌿 If you plan to exercise in the evening, put on your workout clothes as soon as you get home from work or from running errands. Do you really want to take them off without making them sweaty first? This strategy has helped many of my patients move from "too tired to exercise" to actual exercise.

🌿 If you spend your days at home, leave a yoga mat or some hand weights in a conspicuous place.

🌿 Each Sunday, plan your workouts for the week. Put them on the calendar like any other appointment. The same way meal planning requires you to look ahead at schedules and obstacles (see Chapter 2), exercise "appointments" must also be planned with your other obligations in mind. When possible, identify a time when you are least likely to get distracted or called away. For me, it is first thing in the morning before email, phone calls, and work get in my way.

- Set the alarm on your computer, phone, or watch to ring two or three times daily for 10-minute exercise breaks.

- Commit to working out with a buddy. Pick someone you really don't want to disappoint.

- Send yourself an email reminder with an encouraging statement such as "I love how I feel after a good workout" or "I'll find time for exercise now because I don't want illness to take up time later."

Health-Boosting Strategy #45

Give yourself white space.

Before studying nutrition, I took communications courses in college. I learned about white space—the deliberate absence of content. Compared to a crowded or cluttered advertisement, an ad with lots of white space says "classy" or "simple" or "luxury." In a book or on a webpage, having ample white space keeps the eye focused on the words. A page of solid text broken up with lots of white space in appropriate places with bullets and lists is less intimidating than solid text.

I need white space in my life. It's much easier to enjoy my meal when I'm surrounded with white space—a lack of noise (phone, TV, dogs barking), lack of clutter (mail, stacks of magazines, dirty dishes, backpacks, and textbooks), and lack of competing obligations (answering emails, reading newsletters, talking on the phone). Creating space in your mind and in your life gives you room to be creative, problem solve, and feel grounded. At least it does for me. If you've ever felt that your best ideas come to you when you're on a long drive, in the shower, or walking in the park, then you have appreciated white space. If you've recently said that you're desperate for breathing room, what you're craving is white space.

The busier and more overworked you are, the less likely you are to give yourself white space because you are forever multitasking and filling every minute with some important task. Yet giving yourself this white space can make you more efficient, more balanced, and happier. Some people meditate. Others find calm in yoga. My white space is my morning jog. I don't think about jogging. I don't plan to think about anything, really. But by the time I'm back home, I've planned my day, remembered something important that was about to be neglected, solved a problem or two, and I am much more prepared to start my day.

So carve out some white space for yourself. It will help you to find the energy and motivation to build the skills described in this book, as well as offer you space for greater creativity, problem solving, and a sense of calm.

ᘞ Getting Started Tips

ᘞ What are examples of white space that you've enjoyed before?

ᘞ What brings you a feeling of peace?

ᘞ What techniques help you deal with stress?

Once you've answered these questions, ask yourself what your barriers are to taking white space and how you can overcome them. White space can be as long or as short as you want it to be and taken as often as you feel you need it. I have taken mine nearly every day for more than two decades. Luckily for me, it doubles as exercise.

Health-Boosting Strategy #46

Snooze your way to better health.

Like many people, I'm tempted to skimp on sleep when I feel overly busy. I find, though, that it is almost always counterproductive. It may sound strange that sleeping can actually help you save time, but it can. When we are sleep deprived, we are inefficient, more apt to make time-sucking mistakes, and more likely to get sick. Without a doubt, adequate sleep is as important to health as diet and regular physical activity. Inadequate sleep is linked to weight gain, reduced insulin sensitivity (even in people without diabetes), more heart disease, reduced immune function, and other problems, including being grumpy. And if you're sleepy and aggravated, you're much less likely to be motivated to eat well, exercise, and put energy into learning new things.

Get a good night's rest. These guidelines should help:

- Schedule a bedtime and do your best to stick with it. When possible, get up at approximately the same time each day.

- Exercise regularly. Many people find it hard to relax for bed if they've engaged in vigorous activity in the previous few hours. Try to schedule your exercise earlier in the day if possible. Yoga in the evening may actually help you, however.

- Avoid caffeine, alcohol, and large meals several hours before bed. Alcohol might help you get to sleep, but it will disrupt your sleep shortly thereafter. If you're not sleeping well, drinking alcohol is a big mistake.

- Make your bedroom an ideal place to sleep. A cool room helps some people sleep better. Consider using a fan. Your room should also be quiet (sometimes I wear earplugs) and dark.

- Establish a bedtime ritual. Enjoy a cup of decaf tea, take a relaxing bath, read a book, listen to soothing music, meditate, or practice yoga. Following the same routine night after night helps set the stage for a sound slumber.

- Keep worries out of bed. I know this is hard. The busier and more overworked we are, the more apt we are to worry about all the things that haven't gotten done. I also know that problems seem far worse in the middle of the night. I learned a trick years ago to help me deal with the nuisance of fretting instead of sleeping. If you practice it often, it will probably work for you too. In my mind, I visualize putting my worry in a place where I can find it and work on it in the morning. I remind myself that it's waiting for me and that I can deal with it at an appropriate time. It amazes me how well this technique has worked.

- Call the doc. If none of these bedtime adaptations works or if you sleep but rarely feel rested, a visit to the doctor's office is in order.

You may also enjoy using a sleep tracker. There are several good ones on the market. I use the Flex™ Wireless Activity and Sleep Wristband by Fitbit. It wasn't until I started using it that I realized I wasn't allowing myself adequate time to sleep. Seven hours in bed wasn't enough because I wasn't sleeping from the minute my head hit the pillow until the alarm woke me. It takes time to fall asleep, plus I often wake in the middle of the night at least once. Flex™ gives me a chart identifying when I get up to use the bathroom and when I'm tossing and turning. It's an interesting chart that has shown me I need at least 7 1/2 hours in bed to get 7 hours of sleep. Other sleep trackers include:

- Jawbone UP™: similar to the Flex™

- Sleep Cycle: an iPhone app

- SleepBot: an Android app

Health-Boosting Strategy #47

Stand, don't sit.

Being physically active for 30–60 minutes each day hugely improves health. What you do the other 23 hours each day is also critical. Recent studies have shown that sitting for long periods of time is linked to increased health problems, including a higher risk for cancers of the colon, endometrium, ovary, and prostate as well as insulin resistance, abnormal cholesterol levels, and obesity. The good news is that very short breaks in sitting are associated with health improvements such as reduced markers of inflammation.

I love my solution to the problem of sitting too long. I got a treadmill desk! There are many versions of walking stations. A search on YouTube shows you a variety of ready-made desk/treadmill combinations and homemade desks to fit over treadmills. I bought the TrekDesk that fits with my treadmill. You can see a video of me here: https://www.youtube.com/watch?v=l8QBju_Q7u8.

Some other ideas to be active in addition to your formal exercise program:

- Set an alarm to get up every hour for 1 or 2 minutes. Stand, stretch, do calf raises, or do push-ups against a wall. It doesn't matter; just get up.

- Use the bathroom on the floor one level above or below you.

- Let the dog out instead of asking a family member do it.

- Walk the dog.

- Play with the kids or grandkids.

- Hunt for shells instead of sitting on the beach.

- Garden.

- Hide the remote control from yourself.

- Do 30 seconds of any exercise before each meal.

Health-Boosting Strategy #48

Don't confuse urgent with important.

The common mistake of confusing urgent with important makes busy people busier and more stressed out.

The phone is ringing. A client and your sister both just sent you an email, and a follower tweeted you. Your neighbor asks if you'll run over to feed the cats while she's away. Each of these interruptions could potentially distract you from tasks of greater importance. When you're feeling overwhelmed by the length of your to-do list or lack of progress on big goals, take a step back to see if you are emphasizing things that are important, not things that are urgent but of little importance. You might be spending more time on urgent, unimportant tasks than you think you are.

In his book, *The 7 Habits of Highly Effective People*, Stephen Covey introduced the Urgent/Important Matrix. Things that we spend time on fall into one of four categories:

BOTH URGENT AND IMPORTANT: Ignoring a warning light on your car can cost you thousands of dollars, so you truly need to tend to this quickly. Your child has a fever, so you need to drop everything to take her to the doctor.

NOT URGENT, BUT IMPORTANT: Exercise, meditation, meal planning, stocking your pantry with healthful and quick-to-prepare foods, planning ahead for work or other deadlines, power washing the house, and reading to your children are all very important, but none requires your immediate attention.

URGENT, BUT NOT IMPORTANT: A stranger comes to your door asking you to sign a petition. You get up right away because the doorbell rings, not because this petition is important to you.

NEITHER URGENT NOR IMPORTANT: Neither Internet surfing nor paging through a boring magazine qualifies as important or urgent.

Covey suggested that we spend more time working on things in the second category— important, but not urgent. I agree. I see my busiest patients tempted to skip exercise class or order takeout when they have an abundance of nonurgent emails and calls to tend to or because they have important matters that arose from lack of planning. Let's spend more time on managing stress, engaging in activities that make us happy, planning and preparing meals, exercising, sleeping, and getting organized for home renovations or big work projects. Not only will we be healthier and have fewer urgent problems related to health, but we'll have fewer urgent matters of other types too, because we will have planned ahead and built a solid foundation for our work, relationships, and other obligations. The car is less likely to flash a warning light because we have kept up with routine maintenance. We won't rush around to find something for dinner because we have carefully stocked the pantry and freezer.

And we aren't frantically trying to finish a report before a deadline because we failed to plan ahead. Learn more in *The 7 Habits of Highly Effective People*.

✌Getting Started Tips

Each morning, look at your to-do list. Prioritize the important. Devote adequate time to those tasks that are important even if they are not urgent. Try to stay away from the unimportant ones as much as possible—even if they seem urgent. Each month, consider those important, nonurgent tasks that have never made it to your to-do list. Then schedule that party, investigate going back to school, or finally learn to play the piano.

Health-Boosting Strategy #49

Identify barriers to success. Then plan your attack.

Whether your health goals include managing blood glucose, sleeping 7–8 hours nightly, losing weight, building muscle mass, boosting energy, or anything else, you will always face obstacles. Perhaps your daughter is in a basketball tournament during the dinner hour, or you have an upcoming business trip or a time-consuming volunteer project. There are an infinite number of potential obstacles in your future.

Overcoming obstacles means planning ahead, wearing your creativity hat, and being open-minded. Some obstacles cannot be anticipated, but most can be. Some will occur over and over—like having a sick child or getting stuck in traffic—so if you cannot anticipate them, you will at least get accustomed to dealing with them.

STEP 1: Anticipate potential obstacles. Look ahead at your calendar. Anticipate any activities that might get in your way, such as a dinner meeting or the gym closing early, and ask yourself how that activity might derail your efforts. A dinner meeting might mean that you will not be able to eat until a late hour when you'll likely be extremely hungry. Or perhaps it means that you will be served foods that might not be good for you or large portions of very tempting foods. If your gym closes early, it might leave you without a place to exercise or mean that you'll need someone else to take care of your children while you exercise early.

STEP 2: Identify your options. Perhaps you could take a walk in your neighborhood or dust off an old exercise DVD as an alternative to going to the gym. And could you eat before your meeting, or have a small snack so that you can eat less of the unhealthful foods served? There are usually multiple options, some good, some not so good. By being open-minded to the solution, you will surely find one that is appropriate.

STEP 3: Pick a solution and list the steps to put it into action. For example, if your plan is to eat a snack prior to your dinner meeting, you will need to choose what to eat, buy it or prepare it, and carry it with you.

STEP 4: After putting your plan into action, evaluate what worked and what did not. Identify what, if anything, you will do differently next time.

Research has demonstrated a relationship between developing problem-solving skills and success in losing weight. But I've seen for myself how important problem-solving skills are for reaching all types of health goals. Developing problem-solving skills takes practice. At first, you may not even remember to look for potential obstacles. I try to do this on both a weekly and daily basis. Some people feel silly going through Step 2, and so they fail to identify more than one or two possible solutions. The more hectic your life is, the more you need these skills.

Health–Boosting Strategy #50

Move forward with a pro/con sheet.

Motivation is a funny thing. One day you have it; the next day it's gone. I've watched this phenomenon in both others and myself. Do you find that you want something very badly yet you stay stuck in the same place, or that you move forward one step and move backward another? This happens because there is a cost to every change we make. So if, for example, you are motivated to exercise daily to help prevent type 2 diabetes and heart disease, you may also be motivated to skip exercise because it's time-consuming or because it means asking someone else to pick up your children from school. The result is ambivalence and a failure to change.

It takes some work to get unstuck. Explore your reasons to change and your reasons not to change. Ask yourself what are the pros and cons of doing something versus not doing it. You may be surprised by what you learn about yourself. Simply making your lists of pros and cons may be enough to move you in the right direction. If not, you may also need to change or eliminate a con or two. Can you acquire new cooking skills, hire help, or delegate chores to free up time? Will it help to purchase exercise equipment, or work through relationship issues? Look at everything standing in your way, because every con you eliminate makes it easier for you to get unstuck.

Make a pro/con chart like the one below for each area in which you feel stuck. A chart can focus on a broad goal like changing your diet, or a narrow one like eating vegetables with dinner or getting to bed earlier.

PROS If I change my diet …	CONS If I change my diet …
I'll lose weight.	I won't be able to eat my favorite foods all the time.
I'll have more energy.	I'll have to cook more and that takes up time.
I'll make Tom happy and he will worry less about my health.	I'll have to plan my meals.
I'll be able to wear more fashionable clothes.	I don't know what I'd eat when we hang out with our friends.
I'll lower my blood pressure and cholesterol.	They might complain if I don't eat what they eat.
I'll help prevent type 2 diabetes and other health problems.	The kids might feel deprived if I stop baking so much.
I'll feel proud of myself.	I'll have to buy new clothes.
I'll have less heartburn and maybe I'll be able to get off my heartburn medicine.	I'm uncomfortable when people compliment me about my looks.
	I'll constantly worry about gaining weight back.

Additional Reading

AHA Scientific Statement: Fish consumption, fish oil, omega-3 fatty acids, and cardiovascular disease. *Circulation* 2002;106:2747–2757

American Institute for Cancer Research: Foods that fight cancer: garlic, 2011. Available at http://www.aicr.org/foods-that-fight-cancer/foodsthatfightcancer_garlic.html. Accessed 28 July 2013

American Institute for Cancer Research: Learn about colorectal cancer, 2013. Available at http://www.aicr.org/learn-more-about-cancer/colorectal-cancer. Accessed 28 August 2013

American Institute for Cancer Research: Preventing Endometrial Cancer Fact Sheet, 2013. Available at http://www.aicr.org/assets/docs/pdf/fact-sheets/endometrial-fact-sheet.pdf

Harris WS, Mozaffarian D, Rimm E, et al.: Omega-6 fatty acids and risk for cardiovascular disease: a science advisory from the American Heart Association Subcommittee of the Council on Nutrition, Physical Activity, and Metabolism; Council on Cardiovascular Nursing; and Council on Epidemiology and Prevention. *Circulation* 2009;119:902–907

International Food Information Council: IFIC Protein and Health Fact Sheet, 2011. Available at http://www.foodinsight.org/Content/3840/IFIC_ProteinFactSheet_FINAL.pdf

Lally P, van Jaarsvend CHM, Potts HWW, Wardle J: How are habits formed: modeling habit formation in the real world 2010. http://onlinelibrary.wiley.com/doi/10.1002/ejsp.674/abstract

U.S. Department of Agriculture: Why is it important to eat fruit? http://www.choosemyplate.gov/food-groups/fruits-why.html

U.S. Department of Agriculture Agricultural Research Service: Best ways to clean kitchen sponges. Available at http://www.ars.usda.gov/is/pr/2007/070423.htm

U.S. Department of Agriculture and U.S. Department of Health and Human Services. *Dietary Guidelines for Americans*, 2010. 7th ed. Washington, DC: U.S. Government Printing Office, 2010. http://www.health.gov/dietaryguidelines/dga2010/DietaryGuidelines2010.pdf

U.S. Food and Drug Administration: Fresh and frozen seafood: selecting and serving it safely, 2013. Available at http://www.fda.gov/food/resourcesforyou/consumers/ucm077331.htm. Accessed 15 August 2013

Wansink B: *Mindless Eating: Why We Eat More Than We Think*. New York, NY, Bantam Books, 2006

Appendix

GROCERY LIST: Modify this to fit your needs or the layout of your supermarket.

Fresh produce	
Dairy	
Fresh meats & fish	
Frozen foods	
Canned goods	
Breads, crackers, & cereals	
Pasta, rice, & grains	
Packaged fish, soups, & nuts	
Oil, condiments, herbs, & spices	
Other	

Mix-and-Match Weekly Menu Planner

Fill in the necessary amounts of entrées, starches, and vegetables. Add additional items, including foods for lunch, if desired.

Entrées	
Starches	
Nonstarchy vegetables	
Other	

Mix-and-Match Weekly Menu Planner

Example

Entrées	Salmon
	Rotisserie chicken
	Black beans & rice
	Spaghetti & meat sauce
	Oven-fried tilapia
	Cheese & veggie Paninis
	Chicken & veggie stir-fry
Starches	Wheat berries
	Red potatoes
	Sweet potatoes
	Brown rice medley
Nonstarchy vegetables	Salad vegetables in season
	Any 5 or more fresh/frozen vegetables
Other *For lunches*	Yogurt
	Fruit
	Raw veggies
	Hummus
	Lunch meat
	Whole-grain bread
	Canned lentil soup

Detailed Weekly Menu Planner

Fill in your plans for each dinner. If desired, do the same for each lunch and breakfast.

Weekly Menu Planner			
SUN			
SAT			
FRI			
THURS			
WED			
TUES			
MON			
	D	L	B

Detailed Weekly Menu Planner

Example

Weekly Menu Planner

	MON	TUES	WED	THURS	FRI	SAT	SUN
D	Black beans & rice Green beans Salad	Cheese & veggie Panini Salad	Spaghetti & meat sauce Zucchini Salad Clementines	Oven-fried tilapia Broccoli w/ Parmesan Wheat berries Pineapple	Chicken w/ artichokes Roasted potatoes Spinach Salad	Out to dinner	Tarragon Chicken in parchment Salad Strawberries
L							
B							

Weekly Plate Method Planner

Use this chart to help you plan balanced dinners with lots of variety and appropriate portions. You can use it for lunch as well, if desired.

MONDAY		
1/4 Plate Lean Meat or Other Protein	1/4 Plate Grain or Starchy Vegetable	1/2 Plate Nonstarchy Vegetable

TUESDAY		
1/4 Plate Lean Meat or Other Protein	1/4 Plate Grain or Starchy Vegetable	1/2 Plate Nonstarchy Vegetable

WEDNESDAY		
1/4 Plate Lean Meat or Other Protein	1/4 Plate Grain or Starchy Vegetable	1/2 Plate Nonstarchy Vegetable

THURSDAY		
1/4 Plate Lean Meat or Other Protein	1/4 Plate Grain or Starchy Vegetable	1/2 Plate Nonstarchy Vegetable

Weekly Plate Method Planner

FRIDAY		
1/4 Plate Lean Meat or Other Protein	1/4 Plate Grain or Starchy Vegetable	1/2 Plate Nonstarchy Vegetable

SATURDAY		
1/4 Plate Lean Meat or Other Protein	1/4 Plate Grain or Starchy Vegetable	1/2 Plate Nonstarchy Vegetable

SUNDAY		
1/4 Plate Lean Meat or Other Protein	1/4 Plate Grain or Starchy Vegetable	1/2 Plate Nonstarchy Vegetable

Index

vegetarian diet, 64
vinegar, 17
vision loss, 66
vitamin, 105
vitamin C, 60

W

walking, 113–115
Wansink, Brian, 75, 78–79, 82, 91
water, 73–74
Webb, Robyn, *Diabetic Meals in 30
    Minutes—Or Less!*, 42
weekly menu planner, 134–135
weekly plate method planner, 136–139
Weeknight Wonders (Krieger), 43
weight control, 94, 115
white space, 119–120
whole grain, 16, 69–71, 84. *See also under
    specific type*
Whole Grain Stamp, 70–71
Whole Grains Council, 69–71
willpower, 46
wine, 106
Wine-Trax, 82
World Cancer Research Fund, 55
World Health Organization (WHO), 103
worry, 121

Y

yeast, 110
yogurt, 17, 56, 65, 68, 79–81, 86, 89, 95

Z

zeaxanthin, 66
Ziplist, 11